Visceral Perception

Understanding Internal Cognition

THE PLENUM SERIES IN
BEHAVIORAL PSYCHOPHYSIOLOGY AND MEDICINE

Series Editor: William J. Ray
Pennsylvania State University
University Park, Pennsylvania

A Continuation Order Plan is available for this series. A continuation order will bring delivery of each new volume immediately upon publication. Volumes are billed only upon actual shipment. For further information please contact the publisher.

Visceral Perception

Understanding Internal Cognition

György Ádám

Eötvös Loránd University
Budapest, Hungary

Foreword by

James W. Pennebaker

The University of Texas at Austin
Austin, Texas

PLENUM PRESS • NEW YORK AND LONDON

Library of Congress Cataloging-in-Publication Data

On file

ISBN 978-1-4419-3290-7

© 2010 Plenum Press
A Division of Plenum Publishing Corporation
233 Spring Street, New York, N.Y. 10013

http://www.plenum.com

10 9 8 7 6 5 4 3 2 1

Foreword

Almost 20 years ago, I came across a relatively short book by a Professor György Ádám entitled *Perception, Consciousness, Memory: Reflections of a Biologist* (Plenum Press, 1980) while strolling through the University of Virginia library. Because the title was intriguing, I pulled it from the shelf to get an idea of the topic. Within minutes, this Hungarian physician/biologist/psychologist/philosopher had captivated me. Years later, I found myself in Budapest talking with a group of social psychologists. I mentioned to my hosts that, years earlier, I had read a book by a Professor Ádám — had they ever heard of him? The group turned reverential and solemnly noted that yes, even though he had retired, he was still one of the most eminent and active researchers in the country. Phone calls were made and I was soon sitting in his office surrounded by a library of books in Hungarian, Russian, German, French, and English. As soon as we began speaking, I understood why I was so influenced by his writing.

In the fields of psychology and medicine, we come across intellectual leaders occasionally, those with remarkable breadth and creativity even less frequently, and scholarly giants rarely. For the second half of the twentieth century, Professor Ádám has risen to near-giant status through his remarkably insightful and thorough work on visceral perception. In many ways, this book is one of the crowning achievements in his illustrious career. Relying on dozens of his own studies together with research projects in Russia, Europe, and North America, Ádám provides a refreshing new understanding of visceral perception.

How individuals perceive and use information from their cardiovascular, respiratory, gastrointestinal, and urogenital organs has never been well understood. Traditionally, many physiologically oriented researchers have assumed that visceral feedback was relatively automatic and served as an internal homeostatic process. More recently, social and cognitively oriented researchers have hinted that feedback from the viscera was generally of such poor quality that most of the information from that area was shaped and often distorted through basic perceptual biases. Because Ádám's career has explored both traditions, he is the first to my knowledge to integrate the two in such a way that both perspectives benefit.

A good starting point is to compare the way we process visual information through the eye with the ways we use and detect visceral cues from the body. Each retina is made up of millions of receptors that are sensitive to specific light frequencies. Sudden increases in light intensity (e.g., by looking away from the light) can influence the perceiver's behavior and the diameter of the pupil — even without the awareness of the perceiver. In many ways, we can think of the visceral organs as crude eyes as well. The density of receptor cells is remarkably low, and the types of information to which the various systems are sensitive vary from organ to organ. As with pupillary changes in the eye, many of the visceral receptors have the ability to directly influence the perceiver's physiological activity and overt behavior — generally without the perceiver's knowledge. And just as the firing of the receptors in the retina can result in a perceptual image, a pattern of firing of visceral receptors can create a feeling or sensory "image."

Ádám's work reveals some fascinating — and, on occasion, unsettling — problems surrounding our understanding of consciousness. Visceral perception, as he ably demonstrates, is largely outside of awareness. Further, bringing it into consciousness may be both difficult and, oftentimes, unwanted. Consider, for example, one of the ingenious paradigms pioneered by Ádám in the 1960s. A device that can stimulate the small intestine (or other visceral system) is inserted into an individual while, at the same time, brain wave activity (EEG) is continuously measured. Moderate levels of intestinal stimulation will initially bring about immediate changes in EEG, even though the person may not report feeling anything. Using variations of this technique, Ádám escorts us through several studies indicating that intestinal and/or colonic stimulation may influence mood — both positively and negatively depending on the location and magnitude of the stimulus. Also of note is that in some cases people may not be able to initially detect the visceral stimulation but, with verbal training by the researcher, can come to "feel" the stimulation. Indeed, other evidence indicates that learning to control the stimulation may enhance one's ability to perceive it — a proposition that runs counter to many beliefs within the biofeedback tradition.

These findings put many of the traditional emotion theories, such as those of James, Lange, Cannon, and Bard, and even Schachter's cognitive labeling approach, on their ears. Mood and emotion, according to Ádám, can be influenced by bodily feedback outside of awareness. Visceral activity — which can be the result of digestion, exercise, and a variety of known and unknown factors — can thus specifically effect mood states. Note that this observation does not invalidate these traditional emotion theories but points to an important limiting condition to them.

Ádám's research also has implications for work on symptom perception. Those of us who have toiled trying to understand how people come to report a variety of symptoms and sensations have generally assumed that bodily cues are inherently vague and misleading. Indeed, many symptom reports are undeniably influenced by situational factors, our beliefs, and our expectations. One of the problems of symptom reports may well be that they are, by definition, conscious verbal labels. The mere process of tagging visceral cues to language may distort the visceral information.

Possible evidence for the labeling-as-distorting hypothesis is based on research reported by Ádám dealing with cerebral hemispheric dominance and the ability to detect colonic distension among people suffering from irritable bowel syndrome (IBS) versus healthy controls. Basically, the more that IBS patients are rated as verbally oriented, the poorer their abilities at detecting stimulation in their colon. Other work on heartbeat detection cited by Ádám indicates that right-brain (i.e., nonverbal) dominance is associated with better heartbeat detection ability than left-brain dominance. A general pattern of relying on language and, perhaps, consciously analyzing the internal state may distort the normally unconscious visceral perception process.

Particularly intriguing is that this line of thinking has major implications for the study and practice of symptom reporting in the natural environment. The primary reason that humans ever label their internal states is to convey their biological status to another person. Symptom reporting, then, is a supremely social act. We tell our companion that we are hungry or thirsty to signal we want to eat. We label our headaches, pounding hearts, or fatigue to alert our physician, parent, or caretaker that something is wrong and needs to be fixed. We complete a symptom checklist to satisfy the whims of a researcher or, perhaps, an insurance company questioning our neck injury following an automobile accident. Note in each of these cases the verbal reports are intended to communicate information to another person and, in some way, influence others' behaviors. In the absence of other people, we would simply eat if hungry, drink if thirsty, rest or take whatever health-improving action at our disposal if sick or injured. As Ádám hints, if we were alone or without language we might naturally regulate our own behavior based on visceral feedback without ever labeling our internal state — even to ourselves.

It is no wonder that Ádám subtitles this volume *Understanding Internal Cognition*. The visceral information that we are constantly processing ultimately influences our thoughts, language, and emotion. By the same token, social and cognitive processes can shape visceral perception and, ultimately, visceral activity.

As the reader will quickly learn, this is a book that goes far beyond the study of visceral perception. It is a monograph that touches on the central features of the mind–body question and, at the same time, the nature and history of scientific thinking. The topic is as captivating to me now as it was 20 years ago.

James W. Pennebaker
The University of Texas at Austin
Austin, Texas

Preface

I must start with a confession: The leading principle of my scientific life has always been rationality. Of course, for my readers abroad, such a statement seems a banality, but in this part of Central Europe where I live, in the middle of the political, cultural, and economical turmoil of this fin de siècle, witnessing and surviving the immense mass of individual and collective tragedies, the only bonds remained the bounds of reason. A translation into the strict language of scientific methodology would be that the source of my steady striving for understanding phenomena previously regarded as hidden, foggy, sometimes even "mystical," can be found in my endeavor to rationality. It is my strong belief that modern scientific thinking and critical mentality are already able and will be even more apt in the near future to explain yet incomprehensible phenomena and relations. In short, I am an "incorrigible" rationalist in the old, Voltairean sense of the word. Consequently, I cannot accept the views suggested by some contemporary thinkers, e.g., Kuhn (1970), on the relative validity of scientific explanations about the world, the human mind, and so forth. I am unable to regard strict scientific rules and discoveries merely as some transitory "paradigms" that could be and eventually will be replaced by some other ephemeral "paradigms." Such a consequent rationalism led me to my favorite topic, namely, preconscious and nonconscious information processing.

The fate of the signals originating from the internal organs of humans seemed to me from the very beginning of my research career an excellent and even indispensable model of how the brain handles these covert, more-or-less "negligible" phenomena. As I am a physiologist by education and profession, this essay bears the characteristics of an experimental analysis putting some phenomena of mind on the dissection table. Such a disintegration of naturally integrated psychological activities raises the question: Isn't the topic of the book merely an artifact? I will try to deny such a suspicion. Of course, the main line of demarcation between real and artificial functions is situated along validated and reproducible observations and experiments. The book is based on proven and published descriptions and experimental data.

In collecting the literature data and the results of our own experiments, we were steadily confronted with the dilemma so clearly formulated by Pennebaker (1995): "moving from lab to field?" I am convinced that the values of the so-called "ecological" perception standpoint (Gibson, 1979) do not contradict the validity of the laboratory experimental point of view in perception studies, but rather they complement each other: each in its own right. The benefits of "ecological" visceroception research are undeniable: They take into consideration the role of environmental (among others also social) factors in perception and cognition. Clinically, symptom reports can be considered as its ramifications. But, unfortunately, symptom psychology, due to its very nature, mixes different perceptive components (e.g., exteroceptive, proprioceptive, humoral) together. Real life is such: Willy-nilly it intermingles, sometimes confuses hormonal impact with real nervous afferent influence, complex emotions with simple dermal temperature feelings, and so forth. "Ecological" psychologists must make special efforts to separate these integrated perceptions from each other in order to clarify them.

The benefits of experimental "laboratory" visceroceptive research are also obvious. They tell us another, maybe more "sterile," eventually more "alienated" story about the hidden signals arriving from internal "true" receptors of given organs. But such a deliberate "strip" of blended sensory phenomena is an absolute necessity. Without such a farsighted and self-determined delimitation of the investigation of a given perceptual event, the result may slip easily from our grasp. One cannot grasp at once the whole internal sensation problem. It is my longstanding conviction that maximizing would mean minimizing.

My great concern in offering this book to my readers is not at all in presenting some disintegrated, disconnected, and incoherent minute facts and ideas. To the contrary, my anxiety is based on some kind of "all-embracing" feature of the work, since the main unsolved problem intriguing me is the rational interpretation of conscious and nonconscious phenomena. Viscerosensory events are considered merely appropriate tools to approach this crucial issue. Consequently, I feel that I stand somewhere halfway between "pure experimental" and "ecological" sensory psychology and physiology.

This is an essay based on experimental data, but containing also conjectures, provocative guesses, half-proven or unproven hypotheses. For example, I raise the question of the possible existence of "visceral illusions" (p. 149) as counterparts of visual, auditive, haptic, and other illusions and hallucinations, although no one has demonstrated the reality of such mistaken perceptive events originating from the internal organs. It cannot be ruled out that just the careful verification of such suppositions and guesses will unite in the near future the carefully controlled laboratory experiments with ecologically validated symptom inventories.

Budapest, April 1998

Acknowledgments

The idea of writing this monograph was inspired by my American friends and colleagues during several study tours in the United States, first of all by my senior friend, Neal E. Miller, a leading figure in American psychology, and further by my good friends Barry Dworkin and Henry Slucki. I started to write the book during my longer stay in Baltimore under the friendly support of Bernard Engel and assisted by Marvin Schuster and William Whitehead. My fellow Hungarian-American scientist, Robert Stern from Penn State, was instrumental in pressing me toward the completion and publication of the manuscript. I am deeply indebted to all these colleagues. I am particularly grateful to William Ray, the editor of *The Plenum Series in Behavioral Psychophysiology and Medicine*, who took great care of my volume from its inception. I am honored by James Pennebaker, who was so kind as to write the Foreword to the book. Many of my European and Israeli friends and colleagues, first of all Rupert Hölzl, and further Eugene Sokolov, Marc Richelle, Shaul Feldman, and others, animated me in the preparation and completion of the manuscript. I am very thankful for their inspiration.

The research on which the book is based could not have been undertaken without the strong support of my Hungarian colleagues, such as former coworkers István Mészaros, Éva Bányai, Eszter Láng, László Balázs, and others. I have relied heavily on the cooperation of my present colleagues in the Department of Comparative Physiology at the University of Budapest, such as Tibor Kukorelli, György Bárdos, Gábor Juhász, László Détári, Júlia Weisz, and János Fent. In the past years I had the constant cooperation of several leading physicians from different Hungarian clinics and hospitals, such as Péter Preisich, Pál Keszler, Ágota Kovács, László Ritter, Béla Lestár, György Buzás, and others. I greatly appreciate the feedback received on different chapters of the manuscript from György Bárdos and Júlia Weisz.

I wish to thank members of the administrative and editorial staffs with whom I have worked on the volume; without them the publication of this book would not have been possible: Klára Gottfried, Zsúzanna Kirilly, Katalin Sándor, and Mária Primás at the University of Budapest and Mariclaire Cloutier, Tina Marie Greene, and especially Michele Fetterolf Kornegay at Plenum Publishing Corporation in New York. The whole publication procedure was started by Eliot Werner, and I am especially obliged to him.

Finally, I want to underline the outstanding importance of my family in this venture (my daughter, Agnes, and my grandson, Tamás). My wife, Katalin Ádám, was constantly the most dedicated, enthusiastic stimulant and sober critic of my creative work. I am exceptionally grateful to her.

Contents

PART *I*

Theoretical Considerations

CHAPTER 1

The Subject of This Monograph

Phenomena taking place inside the body pass unnoticed for the most part, except extreme or emergency situations, like breathlessness, the urge to void, or pathological changes. On the other hand, these internal events, mostly in a hidden way, can influence our everyday behavior, such as our motives, our emotions, and even our cognitive processes. With regard to pathological events we all experience some dim or not so dim physical symptoms in part also originating from internal organs. The subject of these covert phenomena is a fascinating one. Such inner symptoms, according to classical physiological findings, are initiated either by chemical (e.g., ionic, transmitter, hormonal) or by neural impact, but only the latter, namely, the nervous influence on higher brain functions, will be the subject of my analysis. The humoral effect on behavior, phylogenetically more ancient, in contrast to the neural one, was and still is the subject of a wide range of studies, whereas the latter, my choice, has been a sporadically analyzed phenomenon. Further arguments for my direction will be advanced in the chapters that follow.

This book deals with the fate of the information originating from the various internal organs of humans and other animals, reaching the brain via specific nervous pathways and resulting in

3

several more-or-less well-defined physiological and psychological phenomena. The term *information* is used here in its less restricted sense, as a synonym for message, communication, or novelty of signals. The thorough analysis of these internal signals in their theoretical, especially mathematical or statistical, aspects is beyond the scope of this book, although it will not be possible to circumvent some quantitative features of the visceral messages when it comes to the description of the psychophysics of visceroception (see Chapter 7). But in general I regard information originating from organs innervated by the autonomic nervous system as given factors of classical physiological sensory functions eliciting in addition to well-described homeostatic regulatory responses less defined psychological events. This formulation of my topic embodies assumptions that are highly controversial, and I hope to make them clearer and unambiguous as I proceed to discuss my laboratory's own data.

The major question arises instantly on considering the title of this book and the above line of thought, that is, does visceral perception as a specific class of sensitivity and cognitivity exist at all? My answer to this substantial issue is affirmative, although I am aware of the doubts formulated by some researchers—mainly by neurophysiologists—based on traditional principles about the activity of sense organs. Indeed, from the physiological point of view, according to the Sherringtonian classification of the sensory systems, the sensory impact acts through the physical characteristics of stimuli (mechanical, chemical, thermal, and electromagnetic) irrespective of their external or internal sources. In other words, physiology cannot distinguish among several biophysical–biochemical effects of these different stimulations according to their visceral or somatic nature. The lack of discrimination between external or internal receptive phenomena in physiological experiments is reinforced by anatomical and histological arguments. Thus, morphology demonstrates that the viscera, i.e., the cardiovascular, gastrointestinal, respiratory, and urogenital systems, are scattered throughout a wide array of more-or-less differentiated "interoceptive" structures that cannot be distinguished—even by using the most sophisticated histochemical or electrophysiological techniques—from the sprinkled or clustered "exteroceptive" endings of the skin and other extravisceral elements. The histology of visceral receptors is similar to that of these latter structures, the receptive apparatus of the serous sheets of the pleura and of the peritoneum being a transitional category between visceral and somatic end organs (see Chapter 5).

In this case, what renders peculiar feature and specificity to visceral sensation and perception? It is my main issue and conviction that not in the least peripheral events but exclusively central phenomena characterize this special class of information processing. Consequently, its specificity can be revealed mainly—if not solely—by using particular psychophysiological and psychophysical methods. As in my classification outlined in Part IV of this book (p. 132, Table 3), Hölzl, Erasmus, and Möltner (1996) distinguish five different levels of analysis concerning visceral signals (see Table 1) in which only the first level, namely, the physiological one, was and still is the subject of the well-known classical homeostatic and reflex inquiry. The other four levels of representations to be revealed require special methods of investigation. Our own experimental approach was based on such techniques, which were successful in revealing the double-faced, borderline character of central visceral sensory events (see Chapter 10). Namely, by using psychophysical and/or psychophysiological methodology, the issues are raised exclusively by the professional psychologist—e.g., can the capacity to "feel" the heartbeats be taught or is it an inborn ability? The answers to such questions are found usually by applying several combined physical, physiological, and psychophysical approaches. In other words, in my train of thoughts the inquirer behaves mostly as a psychologist, the problem solver as a physiologist, experimental psychologist, or psychophysicist. This way of reasoning gives rise

Table 1. Functions of Afferent Visceral Signals

Level of representation and analysis	Biological and psychological functions
Physiological	1. Homeostatic
	2. Reflex
Psychophysiological	3. Modulation of general central activation
	4. Modulation of sensory input
	5. Orienting/alarming
Behavioral: nonverbal	6. Motivating (energizing)
	7. Directing/discriminative[a]
Subjective: nonverbal and verbal	8. Regulation of mood, affect, and emotion
	9. Informative/perceptive[a]
Social: verbal[b]	10. Instrumental/appellative

Note. Reprinted from Hölzl *et al.* (1996) with kind permission of Elsevier Science.
[a]Functional levels addressed in the present paper and the studies summarized: sensation versus discrimination (detection).
[b]Verbal communication to others; perception of nonverbal visceral signals by others is not relevant here as it does not utilize visceral afferent signals of the perceiving subject.

to a series of serious objections, the main point of origin of which relies on the conceptual gap between measurable physical–physiological and less quantifiable psychological events.

CHAPTER 2

Definitions and Terminology

One essential way to approximate and to narrow the conceptual hiatus consists of presenting appropriate definitions and creating a suitable terminology for psychological phenomena occurring as a result of visceral information.

It is well known that internal afferent impulses reaching the different levels of the central nervous system by tens or hundreds every second, every minute, pass off unreported by humans. In everyday terms, we are not *aware* of the magnitude of our blood pressure, of our gastric or enteric contractions, of our CO_2 tension. On the other hand, many psychologists equate awareness and selective purposeful reactivity (see Mason, 1961). In this sense, the whole animal world, beginning with single-cell organisms up to mammals, is "aware" when reacting to stimuli of the environment. In my presentation, I will use the term *awareness* in the narrow sense of being awake, in contrast to sleep or narcosis. In this respect, arousal is the starting point of awareness, the process of becoming aware of the surrounding environment. But on the other hand, *awareness* and *consciousness* are not synonyms. Physiologically, the desynchronization of the EEG can be regarded as an objective marker of the state of being awake, but at the same time, it is a sine qua non of awareness. The aware person can be

7

nonconscious of what he or she is sensing or doing. Thus, consciousness is a more restricted psychological state, related to and depending on semantics, most frequently on verbal reports. The conscious phenomena, both sensory and motor, reflect a category of central processing activity that tends to be communicated to other individuals, i.e., they are linked to some kind of semiotics. Several kinds of signals emitted by the organism—both verbal and nonverbal—are conditions and products of consciousness. It is hard to conceive conscious experience without some semiotic tools. Mute persons, as well as other mammals, do not have access to verbal accounts, but the tendency toward some kind of expression being the substitute of words, i.e., a trend to symbolize internal events, is well demonstrated.

We have now come to the proper topic of the present study, namely, the nature of central processing of information arriving from the four main visceral systems — the cardiovascular, respiratory, gastrointestinal, and urogenital. At least three terms are used by researchers labeling the phenomena occurring during the activity of one or multiple channels of the sensory system: *reception, sensation,* and *perception.* Walter Freeman (1981), in a paper based on his own data, quoted and accepted the definitions given by *Webster's International Dictionary.* Accordingly, *reception* is a minute alteration of the end organs, a transitory physical or chemical phenomenon, resulting in a topographically well-defined excitation along the sensory pathway and its central projection. By contrast, *perception* is the integration of sensory events in the external world by the organism, especially as a function of expectation derived from past experience and serving as a basis for or as verified by further action. I shall analyze the problem of perceptual structure in detail below. The definitions summarized above make it clear that reception, in contrast to perception, does not involve awareness or conscious appraisal of the stimuli. Both definitions are applicable for events coming from the internal

Close-up: The Ubiquitous Unconsciousness

In this opening statement I would like to emphasize that, despite being a very long story and possessing a considerable literature in the history of psychology, the unconscious domain has remained up to the present a more-or-less neglected or rather underestimated field of knowledge. Although fractions of data and guesses about nonconscious psychic phenomena accompanied the development of our understanding of the capacities of the human mind, it was not until the splendid nineteenth century that concrete and documented facts and successive impressive theories emerged. Among numerous thinkers of the last century who mentioned nonconscious processes as likely participants of mental activities, von Hartmann (1884) was undoubtedly the first to describe with scientific demands the phenomena falling outside the border line of consciousness. In all probability he was inspired by the ideas of Schopenhauer (1844) and Darwin (1872) on the subject and he is credited with introducing the term *unconsciousness* ("das Unbewusste") in to psychological and medical usage.

When underlining the dominant role of the unconscious in mental processes, one cannot avoid switching over to Freudian principles, since for a long period of time it was a general, although mistaken, view that the unconscious was "discovered" by Freud. Lancelot Whyte in his interesting monograph *The Unconscious before Freud* (1960) pointed to the historical facts, that the general concept of the unconscious was conceived around 1700, was the subject of discussions beginning around 1800, and was "in the air" in 1870–1880. This means that Freud and the Freudians made use of then-"fashionable" ideas of the unconscious as prime mover of some mental functions. They developed these ideas substantially, by employing, among others, the highly suggestive thoughts of Charcot (1888–1894), Janet (1914–1915), and others.

I will not go further in critiquing the Freudian principles of the unconscious, since I, and most contemporary psychophysiologists, consider them to be an outdated and narrow system of views. For many years I have been convinced that we must look beyond those views, all the more so since in the last two decades real scientific attempts emerged with the purpose of describing and defining concretely the boundaries of the unconscious and the dividing line between it and the conscious. Excellent summaries of the relevant literature can be found in Nisbett and Wilson's (1977) review paper as well as in Dixon's (1981) monograph. The common denominator of these two and similar surveys is their cognitive standpoint, which goes far beyond the very limited Freudian positions.

Almost 20 years ago (Ádám, 1980), I tried to outline a critique of the psychoanalytic principles of the unconscious and presented a list of nonconscious mental processes. My enumeration contained "afferent" as well as "efferent" activities of the higher functions of the brain and numerous "central" phenomena too. Among "afferent" events I enumerated "subsensory" stimuli, hormonal influences, and of course innocuous visceral input. Examples of "efferents" included automatic learned motor performances, and locomotor sets. The higher-order nonconscious events not having either direct input into the brain, or straight output from the cerebrum, were represented by "subliminal," e.g., unconscious learning, including visceral conditioning, and by emotional reactions. The question under consideration in that period of the late 1970s was inevitably limited to some physiological phenomena in the strict sense of the term, unavoidably omitting the whole sphere of human information processing, renamed today the more fashionable *psychology of cognitive processes*.

It is an old observation that when people are questioned about the detailed processes mediating the impact of a given set of stimuli on a series of responses, they are unable to report on the sequence of events. In other words, the *process* of coming to someone's knowledge remains unconscious, the *outcome* of the process, i.e., the *product*, or the *consequence* may become reportable, i.e., conscious. This basic finding has been reinforced and documented in several theoretical and experimental studies in recent decades, emphasizing that unconscious processes include deep structures of verbalization, computational events, language production networks, and so forth. The nonconscious course of the processes just mentioned points to the validity of a peculiar anti-introspectivist view, which is even more underlined by the fact that people cannot correctly follow and report on the cognitive processes underlying complicated behavioral acts such as problem solving, choice, judgment, and the like.

The literature on the lack of verbal reports about hidden cognitive processes is fairly rich, and includes data (1) on learning without awareness, (2) on subjects' ability to report on the importance they assign to given stimuli in complex judgment tasks, (3) on subliminal perception, (4) on stimuli influencing problem solving, and (5) on the role of the presence of social environment (other people) on influencing a particular behavior. Among the colorful and considerable literary data on unconscious processing, the facts and the guesses as to the process of creativity are of special interest. Ghiselin (1969) considered numerous essays on the creative processes of several thinkers, scientists, and artists from Poincaré to Picasso underlining that the course of problem solving or creative activity is fairly hidden from the light of consciousness. It is no wonder that different authors (e.g., Bergson, 1914) regarded the type of creativity represented by the term *intuition* as a nonconscious cognitive act. According to these authors, intuition is a fulminant process of creating a holistic mental image from a number of cognitive fragments. The sudden formation of cognitive mental maps or representations from mosaiclike incomplete schemata had been the leading idea of the so-called "cognitive learning" theory since the early experiments of Köhler (1925) on chimpanzees. Consequently, cognitive intuition and cognitive learning principles were converted into paired, almost identical twin conceptions about nonconscious collection and integration of fragmentary information.

All in all, it seems to me that Polányi (1964) was right by arguing that "we can know more than we can tell." It appears, however, that sometimes the opposite may also be true: "we tell sometimes more than we can know." The two statements, each of which seemingly rules out the other, point to the same general conjecture: Cognition and verbalization constitute two distinct entities, which in some instances can be interconnected or even interwoven, while in other cases they develop and function separately. Whereas verbal reports postulate conscious state of mind, cognitive collecting of information does not presume conscious awareness in the course of processing, merely meticulous accumulation of fractions of the given information, even if unconscious. Vygotsky (1960) had emphasized before the advent of the influential cognitive trend in psychology that cognition and verbalization developed separately in the course of both phylogenetic and ontogenetic lines of evolution, crossing each other only accidentally, during human development. Consequently, in the ocean of nonverbal, or rather subverbal, mostly unconscious, accumulation of information, the verbal, i.e., conscious, sphere constitutes merely narrow islands or archipelagos. Hence, the adequacy of our saying: ubiquitous unconsciousness!

In this short essay I will not touch on the issues of dissociation theories, i.e., of compartmentalization of the conscious–unconscious domains (see p. 131) originally formulated by Janet (1914–1915). The treatment of that subject would meet with some difficulties in defining consciousness itself, which would go far beyond the aim of the present note. I would emphasize merely that the information, reaching the brain, undergoes at least *four different aspects* of transformation (physicochemical, physiological, psychological, and behavioral). Most of these representations must be unconscious per se, since the different levels of signal processing apparently didn't need to become conscious in the course of adaptation to the environment. On the basis of the great majority of the data on comparative brain physiology, it seems quite obvious that unconscious cognition had and still has a determinant value in environmental adaptability and survival. Probably we are not far from reality if we presume that the different performances of the human mind, constituting *all* psychological achievements, without exception, are based on *unconscious* (or, as Dixon claims, *preconscious) processing.* Dixon (1981) drew three broad conclusions from this statement:

1. The first is that the mind may react to stimuli that for some reason *do not* reach conscious perception. The responses of such unconscious stimuli may be nearly as varied as those of afferent inputs that *do* reach consciousness. Such unconscious inflows include changes in ERPs and in EEGs, effects on short- and long-term memory, emotions, and even influence conscious decisions, verbal manifestations, and so forth.

2. The second assertion alludes to general principles of biological adaptation. According to these principles, the organisms with the largest capacities for accumulating and storing input from the external and internal environment had the greatest chances in the "struggle for life"—in the Darwinian sense of the term. Consequently, survival depended on the amount of previously stored knowledge, unconscious or conscious.

3. The third conclusion formulated by Dixon concerned the *selection* of the relatively restricted domain of conscious phenomena from the broad and rich supply offered by the stored unconscious faculties. He regards consciousness to be a result of human evolution, and to have emerged following the pressure exerted by the needs of optimal performance in the natural and social environment. For example, every sensory modality, influencing the activity of the brain, has both a "subliminal," i.e., unconscious, fringe and a conscious "phenomenal" range, the former

constituting the large "reserve stock" of the latter. Dixon regards "visceral interoceptors" as the modality with maximal unconscious and minimal conscious representation in the mind (see Fig. 16).

world, but characteristically enough Freeman does not put emphasis on the internal environment.

In the above two-step classification, an interposed step is missing between simple, periphery-induced reception and complex, memory-determined perception. This intermediary sensory phenomenon occurs very often as follows: When visceral receptors send messages to the brain, the messages can evoke verbal reports, but they can also be below the level of awareness and, as far as our data indicate, in most cases, they don't rely on previous individual experience, only on the inborn experience of the species. This is the category of *sensation*, which—in my own formulation—corresponds to the Cartesian notion of *sense experience*. According to Firth (1974), sense experience must fulfill three conditions: (1) It must rely on a psychophysical judgment ("I now perceive such and such a physical thing"); (2) the judgment "derives its warrant from its inferential relations to warranted propositions about the intrinsic character of the accompanying sense experience"; (3) these propositions do not derive their warrant from other propositions, rather they are basic epistemically, i.e., they are "self-warranted." The latter condition means that psychophysical laws must be included among the ultimate premises that justify sensational beliefs (pp. 4–18). Human beings must have *direct knowledge* about their sensations, and, as emphasized by Yost (1974), these are distributed among three "departments" of knowledge, namely, human common sense, scientific inquiry, and analytic exploration of sensory fields. Yost named this direct, immediate source of information processing a *sensum* (pp. 19–39).

I believe that the above philosophical formulations correspond to our everyday physiological ways of reasoning, which have been excellently described by Mountcastle (1980). His definition fits best into the conclusions of our experimental results, to be briefly outlined in this book, and which goes back to traditional formulations in experimental psychology:

> Sensation is that mode of mental functioning referring to immediate stimulation of the organism, including hearing, smelling, and seeing; specifically, it is the direct behavioral experience evoked by immediate stimulation of the sense organs. Sensation is no longer strictly differentiated from perception, but the latter term is used frequently to designate a more complete behavioral experience that may involve the combination of different sensations and their conjunction with past experience in apprehending and understanding the objects and facts we encounter in everyday life. (p. 327)

In this definition, the combination of sensations and the involvement of past experience in perception is essential. To give an example from our studies concerning the cardiovascular system, we have found that when distending the carotid sinus with different intensities of mechanical stimulation, adequate firing rate can be observed on the sinus nerve and consequently a sudden fall in blood pressure is characteristic: the well-known carotid sinus reflex. This is a typical example of reception, which is, in fact, a stretch signal to the mechanoreceptors of the carotid wall sending information to the nucleus tractus solitarius and, further, evoking the reflex response. It can be elicited in anesthetized, even in decerebrated animals; it does not require awareness. However, it steadily functions during the entire lifetime of humans and other animals as the most powerful tool of blood pressure regulation. On the basis of this inborn cardiovascular reflex, conditional response can be elaborated in aware animals (and probably humans too). In this case, the sensory phenomenon starting from the arterial wall elicits sensation, at least by the arrival of the unconditional reinforcing stimulus. We do not know whether, in this particular case, the animal was aware of the advent of the conditional carotid stimulus. Our other human experimental data indicate that most people are able to detect heartbeat; this ability in all probability includes stored past experience. Most people feel their rhythmic heart contractions and pulse intervals via a combination of several sensations: real visceroceptive impulses coming from the sensory nerves of the heart itself mixed with auditive ones coming through the pulses of the middle and inner ear, pulsations of the neck and wrist, skin, and elsewhere. Thus, heartbeat detection is a real form of perception in which several sensations—external and internal—play a given role and expectation, due to the storage of experience dating back to early childhood (see p. 104).

Before concluding this introductory discussion on definitions, I must digress on the problem of perception. As far as I know, it was Kuhn (1970) who introduced the term *paradigm* from the field of grammar into the domain of philosophy of science, in order to determine the most general principles of a given compartment of scientific concepts. The paradigms influence whole generations of scientists, and their changes mean real revolutions in our scientific conceptions. Gregory (1974) has drawn a comprehensive picture of several contemporary paradigms for perception-clustering six groups of them, starting with reflexes and tropisms and concluding with feature analysers and representations (pp. 269–279). As a consequence of his grouping, he renders priority to the notion of perceptions that are hypotheses based on actually sensed and previously stored information (this view having a long history from Helmholtz to Craik) and which are expressed as "phase sequences" of neuronal assemblies in the brain, a concept traced back to James (1907) and expounded by Barlett (1932) and Hebb (1949). In my present work, I accept this known paradigm, as it corresponds and agrees with our own data. Mountcastle's practical definition quoted above, is a popular textbook version of this concept.

Thus, I regard visceral perception as a combination of present and past, unconscious and conscious mental sensory events.

Even if the scientific community agrees with my formulation, we meet with many difficulties on which I will expound in Part IV (see pp. 156–157). One of the major obstacles concerns the lack of semiotics as to internal feelings. Even the Cartesians have emphasized (see Firth, 1974) that "a baptismal rule...requires us to name our sense experiences after the objects that produce them under standard conditions (pp. 4–14)." Visceral input to the brain does not have definite, well-articulated semiotics. Rather it has different verbal expressions of vague, scientifically nonvalidated internal states, which are the results of a long historical heritage.

CHAPTER *3*

Historical Roots and Evolution

The first description of visceral sensation, in the framework of our cultural background, can be found in the works of Greek scientists. Plato (1907) in *Charmides* blames some Greek physicians for not considering the unity of body and mind when healing patients. Along with many other terms in modern science, we attribute to Aristotle (1982) the concept of "sensorium commune" or common sensations, from which the notation of *coenesthesia* was rooted. It is most likely that Oriental cultures (the first being the Indian) had discovered and analyzed internal sensations even earlier as judged by the more than 1000-year-old practice of the yogis, who apparently managed to both perceive and even eliminate internal feelings. But it was not until the advent of modern scientific thinking that the perception of bodily phenomena became the object of examination from both psychological and physiological aspects.

Pavlov (1954) had emphasized the role of the internal environment in controlling behavior. In this respect, he was a successor of both Spencer (1872) and Sechenov (1935). Spencer (1897) drew attention to our internal perceptual environment. Sechenov had underlined "dim feelings" in discussing influences coming to the brain from inside the body. All three pioneer researchers based

17

their hypotheses on the most up-to-date ideas and data of their time. The experimental evidence came later, in our century. Sherrington was likely the first to demonstrate a generalized physiological effect of visceral afferent stimulation in 1899 and Bykov, Pavlov's pupil, elaborated the first viscerosensory learned reflexes in 1926. These two lines of research, the pure physiological "Sherringtonian" and the psychophysiological "Pavlovian" trends, are flourishing today, sometimes enhancing and encouraging, sometimes impeding each other and overcoming major fundamental and technical obstacles. Most Western European research groups in this area, such as British and French ones, as well as some renown Indian physiologists, are successors of the "Sherringtonian" tradition, whereas most American and Russian researchers, furthermore, some workers of Central European laboratories, carry out behaviorally-oriented investigation in this field following the "Pavlovian" line. The behaviorally oriented research was later split into two different branches: in addition to the genuine Pavlovian trunk a peculiar ramification emerged in the United States in the early sixties based on the Thorndikeian "law of effect" and on the Skinnerian instrumental (or rather "operant") conditioning paradigms. Whereas the followers of the classical Pavlovian trend called their theory about cerebro-visceral interrelations "Cortico-visceral Physiology," the adherents of the Skinnerian trend labeled their attemps as "Biofeedback Learning" (see "Close-up: On the Parallel History of Two Successive Psychovisceral Learning Trends: Major Stimulants of Research on Visceroception").

For most of our lives, we direct our attention toward events occurring in the social and biological environment: Human awareness is directed toward external perception and cognition. Consequently, special methods are necessary to reveal the role and importance of the more hidden type of perception, the internal one—the topic of this book. Questions arise such as: Is human perception the result of evolution? Do animals show identical

Close-up: On the Parallel History of Two Successive Psychovisceral Learning Trends: Major Stimulants of Research on Visceroception

Research in the field of viscerosensory phenomena was undoubtedly stimulated both by the influential classical conditioning trend initiated by Pavlov (1951–1954) in Russia (later: Soviet Union) and successively by the highly popular instrumental (operant) conditioning direction in the United States inspired by Skinner (1938) and his followers. Although our knowledge on internal sensory events must be considered to be a product of a very long history of guesses, observations, and documented experimental data, there is no doubt that the clear acceleration of the attention of the psychophysiological research community toward visceroception was due to these successive twin trends. Each displayed some kind of peculiar publicity for a period of about one generation (in the USSR: 1926–1956, in the USA: 1960–1990?). The Soviet direction culminated in the late 1940s and the 1950s, whereas the American one reached its climax in the 1970s and in first half of the 1980s. The overpopularization was followed by feelings of disillusionment and emptiness in both trends, which were geographically and intellectually almost completely isolated from each other.

Two historical circumstances rendered impetus to both trends: (1) the state of knowledge in the medical and psychological sciences of the given period, namely, the pressure created by the relevant and powerful clinical observations and facts about the correlation of pathological phenomena with psychological processes, and (2) the suggestive theories of learning "within reach" in the given period, namely, the Pavlovian principles of classical conditioning in the USSR and the Thorndikeian (de facto Skinnerian) principles of instrumental (operant) conditioning in the United States. Both theories declared their universal validity concerning input and storage of acquired information, and both claimed to be recognized as general principles of animal and even human learning.

The Pavlovian direction was based on the fundamental fact that all animals are subject to the laws of classical conditioning; inborn functions, viscerosensory and others, can be taught under special conditions.

The first documented psychovisceral classical conditional reflex was observed relatively early in Pavlov's original Saint Petersburg laboratory in 1918. His close co-worker Tsitovich had demonstrated conditional vasoconstriction in the dog's leg using a limb plethys-mograph. He associated acoustic stimuli (as CS) with rinsing cold water on the surface of one leg (as US) and recorded the volume changes in the other leg. After several pairings the acoustic stimulus evoked a volume decrease without the application of the cold water. Subsequently, in this and many other similar studies, the visceral response constituted the reinforcing US. Investigations in which the visceral component served as a CS had started somewhat later: Bykov together with Alexeyev-Berkman (1926, cited by Bykov, 1947) had elaborated conditioned diuresis in dogs, in which the rinsing of the stomach wall with water through a gastric fistula served as a viscerosensory CS (pp. 81–99). This visceroceptive conditional reflex is regarded as the historical starting point of a rich series of experiments documented in hundreds of articles and about a dozen monographs. The leading laboratory was without a doubt Bykov's institute in Leningrad, his co-workers being regarded as outstanding scientists of that period, e.g., Chernigovski, Kurtsin, Pshonik, Rikkl, Slonim, Kondradi, Airapetyants, and others. The fundamental monograph was Bykov's: *The Cerebral Cortex and the Internal Organs,* first published in Leningrad in 1941, the second edition in Moscow in 1947. The English translation did not appear in New York until 1957. This book, which had been translated in the early 1950s into German, Hungarian, and other languages, exerted a considerable influence on medical and psychological research and clinical practice in Central and Eastern Europe in those years. All the more so, as Bykov's group had constructed a theoretical framework around their data, by claiming that most of the diseases known earlier as "psychosomatic" or as "vegetative" illnesses have to be considered as "corticovisceral pathologies," emphasizing that cortical activities of learned character may constitute the background of these pathological conditions.

The "corticovisceral" Bykovian trend lasted no more than about 30 years. Its vitality and considerable influence in Eastern Europe decreased gradually after the political changes following the death of Stalin, and the Hungarian revolution, since the monolithic Stalinist dictatorship had overtly supported the adherents of this view, unfortunately thus interfering in pure scientific issues. Consequently, the Bykovian theory was interrupted and appears nowadays as a "semifinished" building with several benefits and results and even more mistakes and pitfalls. Its main merit originating from the Pavlovian principles consisted in calling scientists' attention to the role and importance of psychovisceral interrelations in both physiological and pathological processes and documenting in some far-reaching learning experiments the validity of such relations.

The deficiencies of the "corticovisceral" physiology became evident to many scholars even in the years of its climax. Superficial designs of some experiments, banalities of conclusions, and schematic oversimplification of the underlying physiological mechanisms were characteristic features of some papers generated by those laboratories. In short, extensivity was rather more typical than intensive and deep analysis. Co-workers were rewarded for documenting more and more organ functions subject to classical conditioning. And the overemphasis placed on the role of the cerebral cortex in every learning phenomenon was the sine qua non of the reasoning. No wonder that doubt and disillusionment followed, although the clear-cut scientific issues remained for the most part unsolved and provocative (see below).

A peculiar "reincarnation" of the above-described tendency took place in the United States shortly after the publication of Bykov's book in English (1957). In that period the Bykovian studies were already in a decline in Eastern Europe, but the Western scientific community paid very meager attention both to the prior culmination and to the actual decay of the trend, probably due to cultural, linguistic, and political isolations. The Western "rebirth" of the topic can be regarded as a special case of the "Plutarchian" historical phenomenon. It is well known that the Greek Plutarch (46–120 AD) postulated that under similar historical, political, and/or economic conditions, parallel individual careers may emerge and he tried to document his hypothesis in 46 parallel biographies of famous Greek and Roman statesmen (e.g., Alexander the Great and Julius Caesar). The revitalization of the Pavlovian visceral learning trend in the United States seemed to have some features in common with the above Plutarchian assumption.

The second, instrumental or operant visceral conditioning direction was undoubtedly based on the Thorndikeian "law of effect." Skinner, the most influential thinker in the propagation and perfection of this principle, had declared in the 1940s and early 1950s a peculiar "dogma," according to which only behaviorally relevant functions, i.e., physiological changes that result in movements, are subject to operant learning, contrary to visceral changes, which merely obey the laws of classical, Pavlovian conditioning. This strange view was questioned repeatedly by several workers in different fields of experimental psychology and psychophysiology, but it was not until 1960 that the first well-documented experimental denial appeared: Kimmel demonstrated the success of instrumentally conditioning a typical autonomic response, the skin-conductance ("galvanic skin") change in humans. A considerable series of visceral operant conditioning studies followed, among others, using viscerosensory input as discriminatory stimuli (e.g., Slucki, Ádám, & Porter, 1965). Neal E. Miller's group soon became the leading laboratory working on this topic, obviously not in the least obeying the authoritarian "Russian" style, but in the more tolerant "Western" sense. Consequently, most of the leading scientists in the field, e.g., B. Engel, D. Shapiro, E. Taub, B. Dworkin, S. Siegel, and many others, were not students or followers of Miller, but respected his prestige. This was especially so since he was courageous enough to publish not only his successes, but also his failures in instrumental conditioning of visceral functions (e.g., in immobilized, curarized animals). As for the Soviet tendency, some of the workers in this American school of visceral learning had constructed a theoretical framework, coining among other terms the rather unfortunate *biofeedback* for their methodology; thus, their special journal was called *Biofeedback*, and their series of books *Biofeedback and Self-regulation*.

The flowering of the biofeedback trend is over, having lasted no more than about 30 years, exerting some influence on psychologists and clinical psychophysiologists mostly in the United States. In the late 1960s and 1970s, it was overadvertised in the press and in the medical instruments industry, the unjustified expectations causing harm to serious and careful research and application.

The essentials of the biofeedback trend were analogous to those of its Bykovian predecessor: drawing the attention of scientists and clinicians to the importance of psychovisceral interrelations. Even more than its Pavlovian "forefather," it offered additional therapeutic tools to internal medicine in the form of instrumental amelioration of defective visceral activities. Moreover, its techniques seem to be useful in teaching retarded persons, children and adults, to improve their motor activities, speech, limb movements, and even their creative abilities and skills.

The insufficiencies of the biofeedback-trend were also similar to those of its predecessor: superficial design of some investigations and extensive rather than profound analysis of the underlying mechanisms, probably due to the public's hopefulness of the popular expectations. In addition, the evident influence of some narrowly educated "behaviorists" could be observed from the very beginning of this direction of investigation, who openly regarded the brain's mechanisms as a "black box." Characteristically, N. E. Miller's group, deliberately distant from Skinner's followers, by no means could share this "black box" notion. Seemingly, these small-minded views contributed to coining of the misleading term *biofeedback*.

Comparing the two successive visceral learning trends, outlined above, a series of similarities and points of contact can be made:

1. The theoretical bases of both directions had originated from the leading learning principles of the respective times, namely, from the Pavlovian-Bykovian theories of classical conditioning in the USSR and from the Thorndikeian–Skinnerian theories of operant conditioning in the United States.

2. Both tendencies passed over strong and rich clinical argumentation in favor of the visceral learning principle and both denied the validity of Freudian "psychosomatics," despite making use of the thesaurus of pathological cases and even of the terminology of the latter.

3. Both trends suffered from considerable pressure exerted by public opinion, realized in the form of political influence (in the USSR) or of publicity (in the United States). As a consequence of this parascientific pressure, exaggerated expectations emerged, resulting finally in disillusionment and loss of real scholarly interest.

4. For these reasons, both directions are at present in a "semi-finished," empirical state, having failed at elucidating the main laws and mechanisms of visceral learning.

In the long run, a series of unsolved fundamental issues burden both the Bykovian and the Skinnerian visceral learning trends, which, at the same time, offer prospects for the future. Listed below are some open questions in the broader field of conditioning of the function of internal organs supplied by autonomic innervation. The intriguing character of most of these unsolved problems may arouse the curiosity and motivation of future researchers in related topics of psychophysiology.

Mediation? The basic phenomenon of the learning ability of most visceral organs and systems has been repeatedly documented, but the intermediary and relay structures, as main tools of this activity, are mostly unknown. In all probability, somatic mediation is always a sine qua non of learning, but the existence of "pure" brain–visceral interrelations cannot be excluded either.

Organs and systems? Despite the past 70 years of visceral conditioning research, a more-or-less complete list of internal organs, or visceral systems subject to learning can not be compiled. Actually we don't have any principle of classification of the visceral field apt to conditioning. Although Bykov in his initial monograph, cited above, made such an attempt, his spectrum of organs was obviously incomplete and, as far as I know, nobody has tried since then to determine the border lines of organ conditioning! For example, the production of T_3 and T_4 hormones (tri- and tetraiodothyronine) seems to be subject to psychic influence in the thyroid gland, consequently also to learning, but what about the calcium-regulatory hormones of the thyroid?

Parameters? The general schemes and particular schedules for reliable visceral conditioning are unknown. In the Bykovian laboratories the issue was never raised; in the Skinnerian school, and later in Neal Miller's group, the parameters were constantly on the agenda, but even a rough general schedule could not be constructed. To the best of my knowledge, only Dworkin (1993) has tried to give broad outlines of some parameters.

Short- and long-term visceral memory? The duration of a particular learned and stored visceral change is for the most part unknown. Obviously its elucidation will depend on the characterization of the parameters mentioned above, but at present this entire field is unexplored.

Personality? The relation of the whole visceral learning problem to individual types and traits has to be solved. In other words, the conditioning of internal organs is to the same extent personality dependent as the learning process of behaviorally more relevant functions. But the entire, very complex set of problems is at present in a turbulent state.

Interrelations? The connections between classical and instrumental visceral conditioning in real-life situations, i.e., outside the experimental laboratory, have to be elucidated. In the nonvisceral domain, the Skinnerians made strenuous efforts in this respect, but not in the sphere of learning of internal organs.

Viscerosensory input? J. Brener, G. Jones, and others had postulated that visceral afferent messages constitute preliminary conditions for successful "biofeedback." Much earlier, Bykov (1947) had presumed the same necessity in the case of classical "corticovisceral" learning. But at present the available data are rather controversial, and the role of viscerosensory input in visceral conditioning remains to be decided definitively.

---

sharing of their external versus internal perception? What about ontogeny from birth to adulthood, particularly with respect to learning? Frankly speaking, these are based more on guesses and presumptions than on facts.

Along the animal world's evolutionary line, one can find sporadic data pointing to the major importance of nerves innervating the viscera, in comparison with somatic nervous pathways, in a great number of invertebrate classes from flatworms to snails. In vertebrate species, a similar distinction has also been demonstrated. In a previous monograph (Ádám, 1967), I quoted the few relevant data, such as Barnard's (1936) study of the comparative morphology of the bulbar visceral afferent fibers in vertebrates. The development is closely related to physiological function. In the Cyclostomata (e.g., the lamprey), a cellular organization of the bulbar centers of visceral afferents is almost absent, whereas in the cartilaginous fish there is a marked differentiation, especially in the visceral afferent area associated with the glossopharyngeal nerve.

Amphibians show almost no development in the organization of visceroceptive nuclei; a slightly higher development is observable in the acaudates than in the tailed species. The same holds for the bulbar visceral centers of reptiles. However, birds and mammals show an abrupt development of these centers, both in size and in structure. This rapid evolution must be connected with the vast extension of the visceral (gastrointestinal, respiratory) receptor fields and clearly indicates the strong relationship between structure and function.

Receptors of the gastrointestinal tract in vertebrates were studied extensively by Milohin (1963). In amphibians there is a relatively low state of evolution of the structure of these viscerore-ceptors. In reptiles, however, the presence of encapsulated endings can be demonstrated. Milohin concludes that:

1. In the course of phylogenetic evolution, visceroceptors became more and more differentiated, and at the same time increased in number along the gastrointestinal tract.

2. The development of the central nervous structures is closely related to the development of peripheral afferent endings in the visceral organs.

The morphology of cardiovascular receptors in vertebrates has been excellently summarized, from the viewpoint of evolution, by Ábrahám (1964).

According to the data on comparative physiology, an increase of pressure in the floats of fish, which is accompanied by a volley of discharge in the afferent fibers, greatly affects the movement of the float itself and the function of the heart and lungs (Koshtoyants 1950–1957). Sokolov (1955) was successful in establishing conditioned reflexes from the receptors of the floats of fish.

The comparative physiology of the baro- and chemoreceptors of the carotid and aortic arch has been perhaps the most extensively studied problem of visceroception in the lower vertebrates. Stimulation of the branchial vessels in teleosts led to changes in function similar to those resulting from chemo- and mechanoreceptor stimulation (Kravchinski, 1945). The "vascular labyrinth" of the carotid artery in acaudate and caudate amphibians has been regarded as a primitive carotid sinus (Pischinger, 1934). Stimulation of vagal afferents in the frog evokes a depressor response (Nikiforovsky, 1913), whereas increased pressure in the atrium increases the discharge of impulses in vagal afferent fibers (Neil, Ström, & Zotterman, 1950).

As far as ontogeny is concerned, facts and hypotheses are numerous, although the picture is far from clear. In an early series of experiments on puppies subjected to surgery of isolated Thiry-Vella loops of the small intestines, we showed that visceroceptive classical conditioned reflexes could be elaborated significantly faster than in adult dogs (Moiseeva, 1952). Internal perception of the neonate has been a favorite topic for different schools of psychology. James (1907) emphasized that the infant in the first period of life seemingly does not discriminate external and internal sensory stimuli arising from homeostatic and other changes. For the neonate, these different sensory data are not yet organized and localized; discrimination seems to be a long and complex procedure. The very first phase of this recognition appears to be the tracking of visual and auditory signals by the infant (e.g., preference for the mother). The same idea was proposed by Hebb (1949). These early hypotheses were partially reinforced by Moiseeva (1952), who found that in the dog visceroceptive conditioned reflexes predominate over exteroceptive ones immediately after birth, whereas at the age of 1½ to 2 months, the situation is reversed. That is, information from the external environment becomes more important than that from the viscera. She also found that in the rabbit embryo, i.e., during intrauterine life, stimuli elicited from the visceral domain may inhibit the movements of the fetus.

PART II

Basic Physiological Mechanisms

CHAPTER 4

Conceptual Preliminaries

Adequate Stimuli versus Organ Systems?

Physiological mechanisms of viscerosensory events have been analyzed in detail, beginning with the pioneering discovery of the depressor nerve activity originating from the aortic arch by Cyon and Ludwig (1866). But in our thinking, the viscerosensory system is still not regarded as a special integrated entity of sensory physiology. This circumstance has been vigorously advocated in my papers (e.g., Ádám, 1974, 1978) going back to the monograph published in 1967. But the situation has not changed since then. The causes and the current theoretical trends are discussed elsewhere in this book (see pp. 119–122). In this chapter, I raise this issue in order to set in its proper light the intention to make clear the functions of visceral afferent messages. The first of these relates to their adequate stimuli in their environment (i.e., mechanical, chemical, osmotic, thermal, and so on) in the framework of which they exert their primary impact on the normal functioning of the organism. The nature of the physical and chemical agents exercising influence on visceral afferent endings determines primarily the activity of their own receptive structures and only secondarily the physiological systems in which they act. In other words, the

31

basic principles of activity of mechanical or chemical receptor organs are identical (or at least similar) regardless of whether they function in the framework of the alimentary or the circulatory systems. This evidence is clear to those working in the field of viscerosensory mechanisms, although, to my knowledge, only a few major comprehensive studies have been published in the last two decades integrating viscerosensory processes detaching them from their organ systems (Newman, 1974; Mei, 1983; Cervero & Morrison, 1986).

The Boundaries of the Present Survey

The standpoint of the above major and minor studies in defining the frontiers of viscerosensory function is identical to that of the present monograph: Neither purely chemical impacts nor "quasi"-external effects are included in the limit of our inquiry. I must clarify this double restriction. The limitation on humoral input to the brain seems to be self-explanatory: If we include hormonal actions, transmitter functions, and the like among the visceral afferent, in other words, among "interoceptive" influences, the very characteristic, sharp-featured flow of purely neural messages from the internal organs to the brain would be dissolved in an overall "lukewarm" generality explaining nothing, but revealing well-known banalities about any kind of internal impacts to the central nervous system. Not that the humoral central nervous interactions would have been elucidated, but nowadays it is common knowledge that large gaps plow this huge domain, e.g., the effect of gastrointestinal peptides on the brain. However, this topic is a different, although highly important, story. The object of this essay is literally *the neural information* originating from internal organs reaching the central nervous structures through definite afferent pathways. There is no doubt that in the near future, due to the rapidly growing body of experimental and clinical evidence, the boundaries of viscerosensory events may widen in the direction of special neurochemical phenomena, but at present the necessity of conscious self-restraint of the author seems to be inevitable so as to reveal some rules of this rather neglected field of research.

The self-restraint in determining the limits of this survey must be fixed not only toward the microdimensions of neurochemistry, but also in the opposite direction of macrodimensions concerning sensory modalities on the border line between intero- and exteroception. When Sherrington (1911) proposed his classification of sensory systems into two main categories, it seemed quite simple to determine the dividing line between the two systems, thus, all structures detecting stimuli from inside the body, i.e., "beneath the skin," were called *interoceptors*. It seemed logical to divide interoceptors into two subclasses: proprioceptors and visceroceptors. The former are the structures in striated muscle, tendons, and joints; the latter, the receptors in the gastrointestinal, cardiovascular, respiratory, and urogenital systems. The delimitation of our topic from proprioception is clear and evident, but some problems inside the visceroceptive domain still remain unsolved; namely, the gastrointestinal, respiratory, and urogenital systems are "open" to the external world. This means that a natural steady exchange of materials is occurring through the orifices open to the external world—the oral and anal orifices, the respiratory tracts, the urogenital organs and ducts. The question arises: Where does the visceral receptor area begin and the external receptive field end with regard to eating, drinking, or inspiration? Or vice versa, where does visceroception end relative to expiration, urination, defecation, and the like? In the opinion of the author, it is impossible to give a precise and competent answer to this question. Neither morphological nor physiological background is available for clear-cut delimitation. This issue of conscious (i.e., reportable) and nonconscious (i.e., nonreportable) viscerosensory phenomena is revisited later (pp. 128–133). Let us hope that it will not be long before detectable and reportable visceroceptive events can be separated from nondetectable ones, and such a circumstance will serve as a criterion when more experimental evidence becomes available. But at present, the boundaries of the visceral receptive field can be specified only by conventional agreement among experts in the research area. Based on such a common consent, the mucosae of the oral cavity, pharynx, and larynx are *not* visceroreceptive surfaces, but the wall of the esophagus and of the tracheae are. The anus, rectum, and urethra are supplied with receptors considered to be of viscero-

Table 2. Afferent Innervation of the Main Visceral Areas

Visceral afferent pathways	Origin
Glossopharyngeal nerve (IX)	Receptor zone of the carotid sinus and carotid body (sinus nerve)
Vagus nerve (X)	Receptor zone of the common carotid and brachiocephalic arteries; receptors of the aortic arch and aortic body, heart and pericardium, coronary arteries, pulmonary artery and veins, inferior and superior vena cava; receptors of the alveoli and visceral pleura of the lungs, tracheal and bronchial receptors; receptors of cardia, stomach, duodenum, pancreas, liver, gallbladder, and small intestine
Afferents of dorsal root ganglia (the majority of fibers run in the splanchnic nerve; some of them reach the spinal ganglia and the posterior roots from the thoracic vagus or from the stellate ganglion)	Receptors of lungs, trachea, bronchi, and pleura; receptors of heart muscle and coronary arteries; receptor zone of systemic circulation; receptors of the gastrointestinal tract; renal pelvic and ureteral receptor zones; receptors of the spleen
Pelvic nerve and hypogastric nerves	Receptor zones of the small intestine and colon; receptors of the bladder and urethra; receptor zones of the genital organs

Note. Modified from Ádám (1967).

ceptive character, whereas the vagina is not so regarded, but rather is analogous to the skin of the penis. The delimitation outlined in my previous monograph (Ádám 1967) can be regarded as still valid (see Table 2). This highly illogical and inconsequential delimitation has arisen gradually from medical practice; e.g., the main object of observation and concern of otorhinolaryngologists and dental surgeons has always been, and will always be, the sensibility of the oral, pharyngeal, and laryngeal structures; they were never regarded as parts of the internal environment of humans or other animals.

Visceral pain is also beyond the scope of the present study. In addition to the theoretical consideration outlined above, pain originating from visceral organs is such a hotly and thoroughly investigated field in clinical medicine that including it among innocuous viscerosensory phenomena would be a complete deviation from the aim of this book.

CHAPTER 5

Functional Properties of Receptor Structures

Observations concerning the morphology and elementary physiology of visceroceptive structures began about half a century after the basic concepts of visceroception had been laid down by Cyon and Ludwig (1866), Hering and Breuer (1868), and Sherrington (1899). The reason for this delay can be traced to Langley (1922), who stated—although in a controversial manner—that the autonomic nervous system has exclusively efferent functions. At the turn of the century, even the most respected morphologists, like Ramon y. Cajal (1909), advocated this erroneous concept. The first morphological description of sensory endings in the viscera came from Dogiel (1878), but a long silence followed. Only sporadic papers emerged proposing the existence of autonomic afferent activity (Schofield, 1960). It was only in the 1930s and 1940s that evidence became clear: Adrian (1933) demonstrated different types of vagal afferent impulses originating from the heart and from the lungs. Heymans and Neil (1958) described the carotid sinus baroreceptors whose activity is contingent on the cardiac cycle. Ábrahám (1949, 1964) visualized these cardiac, gastrointestinal, and renal receptive structures in finely impregnated histo-

37

logical preparations. Similar histological analysis was undertaken by Dogiel's followers, e.g., Larventiev (1948) and Kolosov (1956). The decisive evidence on the mixed efferent and afferent nature of the major autonomic nerves was proposed by Agostoni, Chinnock, Daly De Burgh, and Murray (1957) and by Evans and Murray (1954) who proved that afferent fibers constitute more than 80% of the vagus nerve in cats and rabbits. Of the histological classifications of visceroceptors, those of Niculescu (1958) are still valid. He distinguished three types of endings: (1) unencapsulated free nerve endings in poor or rich arborization, found especially in the large vessels and in the endocardium; (2) unencapsulated, sometimes glomerular endings, present widely in the cardiovascular, gastrointestinal, and other systems; (3) encapsulated endings of various types, like the Pacinian corpuscles of the mesentery.

This classification corresponds with the survey by Mei (1983), who proposed two subtypes of simple, free nerve endings: simple branching and unencapsulated endings with rich and complex termination patterns. Most respiratory and digestive visceroceptors belong to the former class; most cardiovascular ones belong to the latter.

It is interesting to note that a contradiction exists between the simplicity of the histological structure and the complexity of the function of the receptors. A careful analysis of the available morphological data reveals that (1) it is occasionally difficult to differentiate receptors from effector structures on the basis of their histology; (2) identical or very similar endings may be found in organs whose functions differ widely, e.g., in the stomach and in the alveoli of the lungs—hence, different kinds of visceroceptors (e.g., mechano- and chemoreceptors) cannot easily be distinguished by histological examination, the differences obviously being submicroscopic or chemical; and (3) visceroceptors are mostly diffuse structures and are not concentrated in organized structures, as are, for instance, the visual and auditory receptors. Visceroceptors form a network of nerve endings in internal organs, e.g., in the cardiovascular system, intestinal system, glands, urogenital organs, in a manner not unlike that of the skin receptors.

Disregarding the morphological difficulties mentioned above, visceroceptors are generally classified in three major and two minor groups, according to the external adequate stimuli toward which they display the lowest threshold, i.e., the highest sensibility: Mechanoreceptors, chemoreceptors, and thermoreceptors are the major categories. Osmoreceptors and volume receptors are often cited in the literature as special functional endings but their differentiation from chemoreception (in the case of osmoreceptors) and from mechanoreception (in the case of volume receptors) is still a debated issue. In addition to these groups, some other peculiar visceroceptor types have been described as sensitive to different modalities (e.g., flow receptors), some of them being of multimodal character. Nociceptors are not included in this classification, pain reception being outside the scope of this book, as indicated previously.

Mechanoreceptors

Visceral mechanoreceptors are heterogeneous with regard to structure and function, as are the mechanoreceptors of the skin, muscles, and tendons. Perhaps the most extensively studied receptors of this group—by classical as well as contemporary methods—have been those of the cardiovascular system.

More than 50 years elapsed between Cyon and Ludwig's (1866) discovery and Hering's (1923) detailed report about the function of cardiovascular receptors. Since then, a vast array of papers and monographs have been published on this subject, a review of which is beyond the scope of this book. For details about earlier data, the reader is refered to the excellent monograph by Heymans and Neil (1958), the bibliography of which includes the principal works on cardiovascular receptors. Heymans and Neil emphasized a point that has been supported by more recent data, namely, that the carotid sinus and aortic arch are not the only regions of the cardiovascular system supplied with receptors. The entire arterial and venous systems contain a network of receptor end organs that play a prominent role in regulating blood pressure and various other functions such as respiration. The conception of classical reflexogenic areas was ruled out by the work of Schwiegk (1935), who demonstrated the existence of a reflexogenic zone in the pulmonary vessels. Besides the evidence of arterial and venous mechanoreceptors, there are a great number of observations on receptors in the heart muscle and in the endocardium, first described by Bainbridge in 1914. The work of Whitteridge (1948), Paintal (1953), Aviado and Schmidt (1955), and others revealed that afferent impulses originating in the atrium greatly influence circulation and respiration. The function of coronary, epicardial, and pericardial receptors has also become clear in recent years. Although the reflex control of circulation has been largely clarified, the extent to which these experimental results helped in understanding the central mechanisms of visceroceptor function remained unclear. An attempt will be made later to answer a small fragment of this question on the basis of experimental data obtained in our laboratory.

The significance of mechanoreceptors in the respiratory organs was emphasized as early as 1868 by Hering and Breuer. A vast literature is available in this field, especially since Adrian (1933) demonstrated discharges in vagal fibers during inspiration and expiration. Three types of receptors are found in the alveolei: (1) slowly adapting and low-threshold end organs which fire during inspiration—they are of primary importance in inhibiting the normal process of inspiration; (2) rapidly adapting receptors firing during expiration and forced inspiration; and (3) very-high-threshold receptors responding only to the maximal forcible distention of the lungs. Afferent impulses originating in the pleura and higher part of the respiratory passage very probably play a part in the reflex regulation of respiration, too. Studying the receptors of the respiratory tract, Widdicombe (1954) distinguished three types in the trachea and bronchi according to threshold; he regarded these receptors to be important in regulating normal respiratory movements as well as defensive reflexes. The J-receptors of the pulmonary blood vessels will be described later (p. 44).

Respiratory mechanoreceptors, such as those of the cardiovascular system, not only control the function of the organs from which they arise, but also induce a number of visceral and somatic responses in other organs (e.g., alterations in cardiovascular and gastrointestinal function). No data are available on the higher integration of respiratory interoceptive input.

The mechanoreceptors of the gastrointestinal tract have been described in many excellent studies, among the most important are Iggo (1957a), Bessou and Perl (1966), and Cervero and Sharkey (1988) (Fig. 1).

There is no doubt that the displacement or the indentation of its membrane is the appropriate or adequate stimulus for every mechanoreceptor, visceral included. That is why, as indicated previously, those endings that adapt slowly to a given mechanical displacement are easily distinguished from those adapting rapidly. Mei (1983) proposed detailed criteria for these two main divisions.

Slowly adapting mechanoreceptors can be found in the respiratory system, as mentioned previously and described by Fillenz and Widdicombe (1972), in the kidney (Niijima, 1971), and in the urinary bladder (Floyd, Hick, Koley, & Morrison, 1977). In the gastrointestinal tract, they have been called *tension receptors* (Iggo, 1955) as distention of the hollow tube is their appropriate stimulus. Iggo (1986) demonstrated that, both in the mucosa and in the muscular layers of the intestinal wall, these receptors are organized "in series." They were first reported in ruminants with small myelinated axons in the vagus and excited by distention, contraction, or compression. Later they were found in cats and other laboratory animals being directed either to the vagus or to the

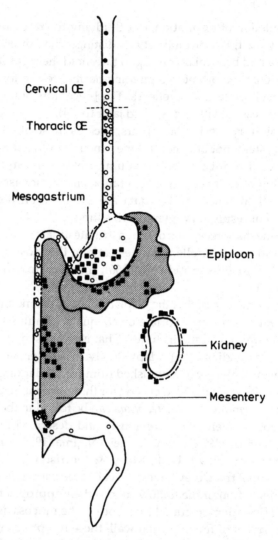

Figure 1. Simplified representation of the mechanoreceptors of the gastrointestinal tract and kidney. The results were obtained with microelectrode technique in anesthetized cats. From Mei (1983). ■, Splanchnic mechanoreceptor; ○, vagal mechanoreceptor; ●, laryngeal mechanoreceptor.

splanchnic nerves. Iggo emphasized that these "in series" tension receptors in the alimentary canal are abundant both in the mucosa and in the muscular layers. This population of slowly adapting mechanoreceptors is linked to both myelinated and unmyelinated fibers, e.g., in the cardiovascular and respiratory systems, but more often tends to have thicker myelinated axons (Mei, 1983). The only difference between these two categories of mechanicoreceptors seems to be the frequency of discharge of the afferent elements. Namely, those with myelinated fibers have a much higher frequency of firing (100–300 impulses/sec) than those with unmyelinated thin axons (5–35 impulses/sec).

The slowly adapting mechanical visceroceptors in all probability can be characterized as special sensors of the long-term state of the given viscus: its distention, contraction, or overall position in the body. Paintal (1954) emphasized that the slowly adapting "stretch" receptors of the stomach are suited for signaling the sensations of the satiation of hunger and thirst.

Rapidly adapting mechanoreceptors, on the contrary, detect quick, abrupt changes in the activity of viscera. Iggo (1986) pointed to the superficial localization of these sensitive endings, being found mainly in the mucosa of hollow viscera and in the endothelial layers of the vascular bed. They do not give sustained discharges to tension or contraction; instead, they are excited by sudden mechanical changes such as stroking or pulsating. Consequently, they are not active in long-term physiological conditions, but discharge to some special situations linked to sudden postural changes or rearrangements of some viscera. The Pacinian corpuscles of the serosa—typical vibration receptors—are included by some authors in this group. The rapidly adapting mechanical endings have both unmyelinated and myelinated fibers, including the largest visceral afferent fibers of A-beta type of the Pacinian corpuscles.

The rapidly adapting mechanoreceptors were described for the most part in the alimentary tract, but they have been demonstrated in the respiratory system as well (Fillenz & Widdicombe, 1972). Their role in the cardiovascular system is not clear, but due to the quick adjustment of the heart rate of the cardiac output and of the blood pressure to sudden changes in muscular activity and posture, their importance seems evident. In general, rapidly adapting mechanical endings are much more difficult to identify than are slowly adapting ones; this circumstance is seemingly related to obstacles in determining the appropriate stimuli that activate them.

This brief and superficial survey of mechanically sensitive visceral endings and their classification into the above two groups according to their rate of adaptation did not take into account the seemingly great diversity of this class of receptors in conformity with their very specific functions in various physiological systems. For example, Paintal (1969) discovered the pulmonary J-receptors in the blood vessels of the lungs sensitive to increased blood flow; Bessou and Perl (1966) described "movement" receptors in the small intestine sensing the displacement of the wall of the alimentary canal; and Hajduczok, Chapleau, and Abboud (1988) detected flow receptors (rheoreceptors) in the carotid wall sensitive to flow but not to changes in pressure.

The synthesis and logical integration of all of these data will be the task of a more detailed overview in the not too distant future. Among the unresolved issues concerning visceral mechanoreceptors is the overlapping between mechanical and chemical sensitivities. Paintal (1973, 1986) had analyzed in detail this double effect by using phenyldiguanide as an artificial stimulant of gastric and lung mechanoreceptors, and for special purposes, lobeline for exciting J-receptors in the respiratory tract. The receptors happened to discharge following both mechanical and chemical stimulation. It is most likely that the excitatory impact of chemical substances on mechanoreceptors is a laboratory artifact. Rapidly adapting mucosal mechanoreceptors, when chemically stimulated, show a rather slowly adapting firing rate (Clarke & Davison, 1978).

Chemoreceptors

This is a collective term designating a group of various end organs with quite different structures and functions. In the visceral field, they have the common characteristic of being sensitive to qualitative and quantitative changes in the properties of chemical compounds. The main chemoreceptors are obviously those found in the oral cavity and in the olfactory mucosa, which form the sense organs of taste and olfaction. However, according to tradition (see p. 35), they are regarded as exteroceptors, and the term *visceroceptor* refers only to chemical receptors of the visceral organs: the cardiovascular system, the alimentary tract, the respiratory and urogenital organs. In addition to these systems, nevertheless, it should be clarified whether certain well-known central nervous structures that have the property of collecting accurate information on the composition of blood and its changes are to be regarded as chemoreceptors: for instance, certain hypothalamic and bulbar structures that accurately and sensitively detect changes in glucose and in hormone levels, and in the CO_2 and O_2 content of the blood. As they lack the high structural organization of the sense organs, these structures cannot be regarded as such; still their function allows us to classify them as chemoreceptors, for by detecting changes in the chemical composition of the internal environment, they give rise to important reflex mechanisms. A detailed description of their chemoreceptor properties is, however, far beyond the scope of this book.

Although the carotid body was discovered as early as 1743 by Haller (1764), chemoreceptor function in the cardiovascular system was first demonstrated by Heger in 1887, who, using the perfusion technique, revealed end organs that were sensitive to chemical stimuli in the hindlimb of the dog. Relying on this finding, Pagano (1900) suggested that the walls of a majority of large arteries contained chemoreceptors. Our present knowledge of chemoreceptor function is based on the work of Heymans and his school. From 1925 to the present, F. and C. Heymans, and their colleagues proved, in a series of papers and monographs, the existence of special end organs in the carotid and aortic bodies, which are sensitive to hypo- and hypercapnia, as well as hypoxia. The reflexes initiated by these receptors, which influence respiration and blood pressure decisively, have been incorporated in classical physiology. The morphology of these glomus receptors was described by De Castro (1928).

Chemoreceptors of the heart, found in the endocardium, epicardium, pericardium, and coronary vessels, form a separate entity. They have received special interest, especially since the debate about the Bezold-Jarisch phenomenon; the mechanism and significance of veratrine-induced hypotension, bradycardia, and apnea have not been sufficiently clarified.

Besides the chemoreceptors of the heart, aortic arch and carotid region, some are also found in the more peripheral vessels, as demonstrated by Heger (1887); since then, numerous investigators have been concerned with this problem, among them Chernigovski (1960).

Except for the chemoreceptors found in the upper section of the respiratory tract, which, when irritated by chemical agents, induce coughing (Paintal, 1986), there is no unequivocal evidence as to the existence of pulmonary and pleural chemoreceptors. Although chemoreceptor-like endings have been found recently also in the lungs and pleura, it seems unlikely that these structures would play an important role in the neural control of respiration or in other functions of the organism. The effect on higher nervous structures of signals originating from these receptors is also unknown.

Much more is known about chemoreceptors of the gastrointestinal tract, as is also the cause for their phylogenetic development (p. 26). This is due first of all to the extensive investigations made in the Pavlovian laboratories. Serdyukov (1899) demonstrated the relaxation of the pyloric sphincter on acid stimulation of the duodenal chemoreceptors. Lintvarev (1901) suggested that the duodenal wall also contained lipid-sensitive receptors. Strazhenko (1904) studied the chemoreceptors of the lower segments of the small intestine. The work in this field was successfully continued by Bykov (1947) and his collaborators (e.g., Delov, 1949; Zamyatina, 1954).

Afferent impulses originating from gastric chemoreceptors and transmitted by the vagus were studied by Iggo (1957b), who described acid and alkaline receptors, and Paintal (1954), who found receptors sensitive to various salts and other compounds. Intestinal chemosensitivity was excellently surveyed by Mei (1983).

Data concerning the higher nervous aspects of chemoreception are numerous, as is true for gastrointestinal mechanoreception (Airapetyants, 1952).

Chemoreceptors of the urogenital tract have received far less attention than gastrointestinal chemoreceptors. In the kidney, the first chemoreceptors of the renal vessels were described by Chernigovski (1960). Chemoreceptors of the bladder were studied by Lebedeva and Khayutin (1952), those of the uterus by Gambashidze (1951), and ovarian chemoreceptors by Beller (1954). The hormone sensitivity of female genital organs and the possibility that nervous structures may play a part in the well-known effects of certain hormones (ADH, aldosterone) on the renal tubuli, suggest further avenues of research on urogenital chemoreceptors. Chemosensitivity of the reproductive organs, the "polymodal" character of these visceroceptors, has been reviewed by Kumazava (1986).

Modalities of Chemoreception

As suggested above, most of our present understanding of visceral chemosensitivity comes from two main bodies of knowledge: the analyses of arterial O_2 and CO_2 detectors and that of gastrointestinal chemoreceptors.

Chemoreceptors in the arterial system are exclusively sensitive to oxygen and carbon dioxide. As mentioned above, arterial chemosensitive endings are mainly located in the carotid and aortic bodies, situated dorsal to the common carotid artery bifurcation and above the aortic arch. Moreover, small units have been found around the common carotid artery and also at some distance from the aortic arch in several laboratory animals (Acker, 1989). The receptive cells of these specific bodies detect the chemical composition and the temperature of the blood *in vivo* as well as *in vitro*. Discharges of the nerve fibers coming from these receptors increase in frequency when environmental O_2 tension (PO_2) or pH falls, when CO_2 tension (PCO_2) increases, or when temperature increases. In addition, these receptors can be stimulated by hyperosmolarity, by hormones, and by several ions (e.g., NaCN, K), but their specificity to oxygen and carbon dioxide is unequivocal. Acker (1989) has reviewed the results of oxygen-sensitivity research, based mainly on his own important data. Having followed the three major steps in oxygen-sensitive reactions—transmitter release, flow changes in the carotid body vessels, and excitation in the nerve endings—he reported that type I cell mitochondria are believed to be the primary sensors of PO_2 decrease, but the oxygen sensitivity of vascular endothelial cells was likewise demonstrated in the carotid and aortic bodies.

Chemoreceptors in the gastrointestinal system are sensitive to a great variety of substances. Their characterization was undertaken by Mei (1983). According to his classification, three major chemosensitive endings can be identified in the alimentary tract:

1. *Glucoreceptors.* Glucoreceptors were found in the stomach and small intestine (Sharma & Nasset, 1962; Mei, 1978). Those located in the stomach and duodenum have axons in the vagus (El Ouzzani & Mei, 1981). Those

situated in the lower duodenum and jejunum are connected to afferent fibers of the splanchnic nerves (Hardcastle, Hardcastle, & Sanford, 1978). These endings seem to be sensitive to any kind of carbohydrate, but their maximal sensitivity proved to be to glucose solution; however, each receptive unit bears a special spectrum of responsiveness. It was demonstrated that glucoreceptors are situated superficially in the mucosa, a finding that reinforces the very early data on the glucose sensitivity of the epithelium of the small intestine.

2. *Amino acid receptors.* Amino acid receptors were carefully identified by Jeannigros and Mei (1980) in the small intestine of cats. These chemoreceptors seem to be highly specific to given amino acids, but nonresponsive to other chemical, mechanical, osmotic, or thermal stimulations. Because the electrical discharges occur quickly after stimulation and can be abolished by local anesthetics, these are superficial epithelial receptors linked to afferent fibers of the vagus.

3. *Acid and alkaline receptors.* Acid and alkaline receptors were first described by Iggo (1957b) having afferent connection to the stomach of cats. Later, similar chemoreceptors were found in the small intestine of cats and rats. These receptors seem to discharge either to strong acids or to strong alkalis, but never to both; consequently, they were termed *pH receptors.* Leek (1977) demonstrated, however, that these same chemoreceptors exhibit a definite sensitivity to mechanical stimuli, at least in the intestine of sheep. Mei (1983) proposed including this group of receptors among "multimodal" visceroceptors.

4. *Other chemoreceptors.* Besides the above three main classes, some authors described other endings as sensitive to chemicals. Niijima (1969) explored liver glucore-

ceptors whose steady firing rate decreases when blood glucose concentration increases. Renal chemoreceptors sensitive to O_2 decrease are initiators of renin secretion. They detect ischemia but not changes in pressure (Recordati, Moss, Genovesi, & Rogenes, 1980). Several papers described gastrointestinal receptors sensitive to cholecystokinin (Davison & Clarke, 1988), which proved to be vagal slowly adapting multimodal endings.

Characteristics and Mode of Activation of Chemoreceptors

The morphology of all of these receptors is characteristic: They are all connected to thin, unmyelinated or myelinated fibers irrespective of their vagal or splanchnic pathways. Their physiology is typical as well: They lack resting activity, the discharges being evoked only by appropriate chemical stimulation. Discharge frequencies increase with the intensity, e.g., if the concentration of the solution is raised. Firing remains steady during, and even after, the stimulation period. The intestinal chemoreceptors are all situated superficially in the mucosa, and spotted stimulation has demonstrated that they possess quite large receptive fields up to 4–5 cm in diameter.

As far as the mechanism of activation of these chemoreceptors is concerned, Mei (1983) considered two alternatives based on literature data: (1) A depolarization and consequent repetitive discharges may be generated by transmitters. This view presumes that the receptor structure is presynaptic to the nerve fiber and that mediator substance(s) can be found in the receptor. This presumption cannot be excluded. (2) The transmitter might evoke a mechanical displacement or indentation of the receptor membrane; this deformation would produce action potentials, as in the case of mechanoreceptors outlined above (p. 41). This possibility cannot be ruled out either.

Osmoreceptors

Verney (1946) was the first to prove adequately the existence of special end organs sensitive to changes in the osmotic concentration of blood plasma. He assumed that the osmoreceptors are located in the part of the brain that receives its blood supply through the internal carotid artery. The endings have not been identified to date; nevertheless, it has been postulated that the osmoreceptors are identical to the hypothalamic cells that secrete ADH. Thus, receptor and effector seem to be the same, or at least located in the vicinity of each other.

It is still not clear whether osmosensitive endings constitute a distinct entity of receptors or whether they can be included in the chemoreceptors. Both the stomach and small intestine detect osmolarity (e.g., hyposmotic versus hyperosmotic solutions) but the same receptive elements are sensitive to isosmotic chemicals as well. This means that osmotic pressure is not the only factor acting on the receptor structures. Mei (1983) emphasized that probably the only peripheral true osmoreceptors exist in the liver. Their frequency of discharge is linearly proportional to the osmotic pressure of the fluid applied, regardless of the chemical nature of the solution (Adachi *et al.*, 1976).

Thermoreceptors

Visceral thermoreceptors have escaped the attention of physiologists for a long time. The few data available concern mainly the gastrointestinal thermoreceptors, and the number of publications dealing with thermoreceptors presumably present in certain parts of the cardiovascular system is very limited: Boenko (1950) described thermoreceptors in the carotid region, and Minut-Sorokhtina and Sirotin (1957) reported the existence of thermosensitive endings in the veins of the skin.

Thermoreception in the gastrointestinal tract was first studied by Simanovski in 1881. His work was continued by Neumann (1906), who evoked movements in the frog's extremities by thermoreceptor stimulation. Thermal stimuli were later widely employed in conditioned interoceptive reflex studies (Airapetyants, 1952): Stimulation of gastric and intestinal thermoreceptors served as conditioned stimuli for the establishment of a series of conditioned reflexes, including differentiation.

These early data were rather neglected and the topic was "rediscovered" in the 1970s when Rawson and Quick (1972) described thermoregulatory reflexes initiated from the gastrointestinal tract: Discharges could be demonstrated in subsequent studies by stimulating cold and warmth receptors in the alimentary canal (El Ouzzani & *Mei*, 1982). The authors in this field of research underline the similarities and differences between epidermal and visceral thermoreceptors: Both categories are slowly adapting structures with an inverted bell-shaped curve of discharge frequency when plotted relative to temperature, but unlike skin thermoreceptors, visceral endings do not display a basal firing at normal body temperatures.

Volume Receptors

The fact that the volume of body fluids is normally held constant suggests strongly that there must be special receptors sensitive to volume changes. It is known that the renal excretion of water and salts is less intensive in the upright position than when lying prone. However, if the neck of the standing subject is mildly compressed, this decrement in excretion fails to occur. This observation led to the hypothesis that volume receptors located in the skull are sensitive to the accumulation of water in the tissues. It is also possible that they are identical to the mechanoreceptors of the blood vessels. Increased afferent discharge in vagal fibers and an increased rate of urine flow on distention of the left atrium also cause diminished secretion of ADH and a drop in urinary aldosterone output. Further investigations are required into the function and structure of volume receptors.

The existence of atrial and ventricular receptors of the heart deserves special attention. In all probability, most of these end organs are mechano- and chemoreceptors, but the participation of special volume-sensitive structures cannot be ruled out. The A-receptors are activated during atrial muscle contraction, whereas the B-receptors are activated during atrial diastole (i.e., ventricular systole). These latter might be identical to volume receptors. Both A- and B-receptors transmit their impulses through the sensory fibers of the vagus nerve to the cardiovascular centers of the medulla. A great number of experimental data indicate that the atrial B-receptors, sensitive to distention, evoke not only rapid blood pressure changes necessary for minute restoration of the disturbed circulation, but also chronic blood-volume changes through the activation of both hypothalamic ADH mechanisms and renin–angiotensin–aldosterone activities. The latter volume regulatory adjustment is the so-called Gauer-Henry reflex.

Multimodal Detectors: The Specificity of Visceroceptors

This brief summary of the literature on the physiology of visceroceptors may appear incomplete to the reader who is keeping abreast of the current literature. This superficiality is due not only to this book's focus on central nervous events related to viscerosensory phenomena, but also to the increasingly popular conception that challenges the principle of specific nerve endings susceptible to specific energies.

Paintal (1954) was the first to demonstrate that the mechanoreceptors of the stomach are also sensitive to chemical stimuli. Zotterman (1953) demonstrated acetylcholine sensitivity of the thermoreceptors of the tongue. The question of specificity is still open: In the case of the dermal receptors, some authors deny the existence of specific receptors (Weddell, 1941). With respect to the visceroceptors, the data are even more inadequate for a definitive answer. In comparing mechanisms, it is especially difficult to decide whether osmoreception is different from chemoreception, or volume reception from mechanical stimulation. Thus, the doctrine of receptor specificity enunciated by Müller (1840) has still not been applied to the visceroceptors, although some new data are available.

It is well known among workers in the field that a class of sensory visceral endings in the alimentary tract discharge markedly irrespective of the modalities of stimuli applied, such as mechanical, chemical, thermal, or osmotic (Harding & Leek, 1972; Clarke & Davison, 1978). Mei (1983) tentatively raised the question of whether these multimodal gastrointestinal receptors are polymodal nociceptors like the pain endings in the skin or whether they are actually nonspecific units. He proposed the classification of visceroceptors in two main categories concerning sensitivity to modalities: (1) specific receptors such as arterial or gastrointestinal chemoreceptors or mechanoreceptors and (2) nonspecific receptors such as the multimodal visceral afferent endings mentioned above. It can be presumed that polymodality of certain visceroceptors is an adaptive phenomenon to the environment; e.g., the arrival in the stomach of food must be signalized to brain centers by both mechanical and chemical characteristics of the alimentary bolus. One circumstance has to be underlined: The macromorphology of visceroceptors does not reveal anything about their specificity, except the Pacinian corpuscles in the mesentery and the chemoreceptors of the carotid bifurcation and of the aortic arch.

One conclusion, however, seems to be certain: The fundamental characteristics of the generation and conduction of sensory impulses are the same for various visceroceptors. The basic properties of sensory end organs have been clarified by studying the receptor potentials of a visceroceptor, namely, the Pacinian corpuscle of the cat's mesentery (Gray, 1959). The nerve ending loses its myelin sheath near the Pacinian corpuscle. The axon membrane within the receptor body has properties essentially different from those in other segments where the nerve is myelinated. Stimulation of the bare axon in this part will generate local potentials, the amplitude of which is correlated with the strength of stimulus. This receptor potential does not respond according to the "all-or-none" law, cannot be abolished by procaine, may summate, and lasts as long as the stimulus is applied. Naturally, in rapidly adapting receptors, like the Pacinian corpuscle, receptor potential diminishes slowly during stimulation. The receptor potential—which is a true generator potential—evokes spike discharge in the adjacent myelinated segment of the axon whenever it is sufficiently intensive to reach the threshold of this axon segment. A spike potential is conducted along the axon, its characteristics determined by those of the nerve fiber. Depolarization in this segment of the axon occurs in the sense of the "all-or-none" law, hence the propagated response is phasic and is characterized by a well-defined refractory period.

The important question of how stimulus energy is converted into a receptor potential has not been answered. It is possible that the mechanical stimulation of the Pacinian corpuscle causes distortion of the concentric lamellae enclosing the nonmyelinated segment of the axon. This deformation, in turn, leads to altered ion fluxes resulting in depolarization of the membrane. According to another hypothesis, acetylcholine liberated in the end organ increases the permeability of the membrane, thereby halting the active transport of ions, thus generating a receptor potential. The initial phase of a receptor potential is presumably not the same in chemoreceptors, yet the subsequent electrical changes, i.e., the receptor potential itself and the spike discharge following it, must be similar for various kinds of end organs.

CHAPTER 6

Visceral Afferent Pathways and Central Projections

The Primary Visceral Afferent Neuron

As indicated above, there is no evidence in the literature that the formation of visceral receptor potentials and propagated action potentials differs from exteroceptive electrical events. Nevertheless, visceral afferent structures display a higher sensitivity to pharmacologically active substances and different chemicals than somatic sensory endings (Paintal, 1986). A number of other significant—mostly morphological—features distinguish the primary afferent visceral neuron from the somatic one, the first of which is the location of cell bodies within the afferent spinal and cerebral ganglia. These cell bodies are not randomly distributed, but rather form marked clusters. In spinal ganglia, these groupings of somata are located peripherally around fiber bundles, whereas in the nodose ganglion of the vagus the fiber packets surround the cell groups.

Before detailing the possible functions of the visceral afferent neurons, I must address an important point that for many years has hindered research in this topic, namely, the widely asserted

57

erroneous view as to the exclusively efferent character of the autonomic (vegetative) nervous system. Interestingly enough, this view is attributed to Langley, who in the opening lines of his book, published in 1922, actually stated that the autonomic nervous system consists of "nerve cells and nerve fibers by means of which efferent impulses pass to tissues other than multinuclear striated muscle." This statement and some others from the same epoch led the scientific community to forget Langley's assertion published two decades earlier (Langley, 1903) about "afferent sympathetic fibers" when this unquestioned authority had mentioned the viscerosensory fibers running in sympathetic nerve bundles. This controversy becomes even more evident if we refer to the early work of Langley and Dickinson (1889) demonstrating for the first time the presence of afferent fibers in autonomic nerves. In conclusion, recent authors (Cervero & Foreman, 1990; Ádám, 1993; Jänig, 1996) emphasize that the deficient view not recognizing the existence of a special visceral afferent system was only a myth incorrectly attributed to, but not really initiated by, Langley.

Let us return to the main functions of visceral primary afferent neurons. There is general agreement among the authors in this field (Cervero & Foreman, 1990; Jänig, 1996) that these sensory neurons are in some respect interfaces between the viscera and the brain, and consequently must have multiple functions. Jänig has recently summarized these possible actions in five points, emphasizing that all five roles serve one main general aim, the protection of the integrity of visceral tissue and the signalization of the actual conditions of the given organ. These five points can be briefly outlined as follows:

1. To encode physical (distention, contraction) and chemical events by centripetal impulses leading to organ reflexes and "distinct sensations"

2. To evoke, via collateral visceral fibers, extraspinal reflexes, mainly in the gastrointestinal and the urogenital field

3. To initiate local processes, independent of the CNS and of the prevertebral ganglia, such as changes in motility, in secretory events, and in local blood flow

4. To support trophic functions, namely, to contribute to the maintenance of the normal structure of the visceral tissues

5. To act as transport pathways for retrograde neurotrophic substances, having long-term effect on the synaptic connections of these primary afferent neurons

It seems evident that the claim to fulfill the role of an interface between the visceral periphery and the brain centers can be assigned only to the first point of the functions listed, namely, that of evoking organ reflexes and "distinct sensations." I will return repeatedly to Jänig's "distinct sensations," which touches the main topic of the present work. The other four points, although highly important, do not need to be analyzed in detail here, as they are too distant from my main interest.

Contrasting with Jänig's classification, Cervero and Foreman (1990) divide afferent visceral signals in two classes, namely, those that do not evoke conscious sensations (e.g., blood pressure changes, chemical composition of the chyme) and those that result in the conscious perception of a sensation (e.g., gut distention, cardiac ischemia). I will demonstrate in what follows the reciprocal transition of viscerally triggered central events between these two classes (see Chapter 10).

The afferent nerve fibers starting from visceral neurons that are present in autonomic, i.e., sympathetic or parasympathetic, nerve bundles are usually categorized in two distinct types: primary afferent fibers and enteric afferent fibers.

The primary afferent axons are similar to somatic afferents having their cell bodies in the spinal or in the cranial ganglia, as outlined above. Their receptor structures are situated in the blood vessels of viscera, in the walls of hollow internal organs, or in the serosa covering these organs. The afferent fibers travel either in sympathetic or in parasympathetic bundles (Fig. 2). Cell bodies of the parasympathetic axons lie either in the sacral (S2–S4) dorsal root ganglia or in the cranial parasympathetic ganglia of the facial nerve VII (geniculate ganglion), of the glossopharyngeal nerve IX (petrosal ganglion), or of the vagus nerve X (nodose ganglion). Cell bodies of the sympathetic fibers are situated in the dorsal root

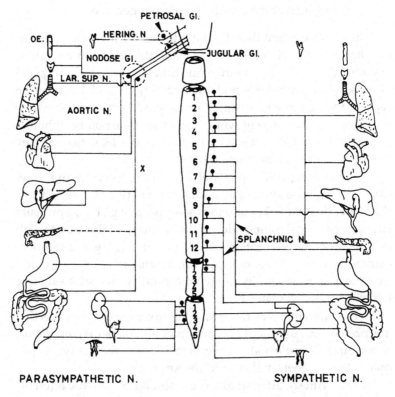

PARASYMPATHETIC N.   SYMPATHETIC N.

Figure 2. Sympathetic and parasympathetic division of the peripheral viscerocep-tive system. OE, cervical esophagus; N, nerve; Gl., ganglion; LAR.SUP.N., laryn-geal superior nerve; X, vagus nerve. From Mei (1983).

ganglia at the thoracic and upper lumbar spinal level. Some of these sympathetic afferent fibers make collateral contact with sympathetic preganglionic neurons in prevertebral ganglia. This collateral connection may be the anatomical background of peripheral regulation outlined in points 2–5 of Jänig's classification.

The number of primary afferents running in sympathetic and parasympathetic nerves is an intriguing issue not generally known even among well-trained specialists in anatomy or histology. These precise estimates reflect painstaking work carried out by several authors (e.g., Andrews, 1986; De Groat, 1986). The numbers have been estimated via tracing methods using different tracers such as horseradish peroxidase, by light- and electron-microscopic fiber counts, and other means. The authors agree on the relatively low density of afferent innervation of the internal organs as compared with that of the skin or the muscles, and on the large differences between the number of visceral afferents in sympathetic and parasympathetic nerves. According to Jänig and Morrison (1986), in all sympathetic nerve bundles of the cat the total number of visceral afferents is 16,000, which constitute about 20% of the total fibers in the thoracic and lumbar dorsal afferent roots. The parasympathetic bundles display a much higher density of viscerosensory fibers. In the cat, more than 80% of all axons of the vagus and 50% of the fibers of the pelvic nerve are visceral afferents. This means that about 40,000 vagal and 7,000 pelvic afferents innervate the abdominal cavity of the cat, a ratio of 1 to 3 in favor of the parasympathetic supply. Less than 10% of the sympathetic afferents are large myelinated fibers connected, according to Leek (1972), to Pacinian corpuscles. The overwhelming majority of such sympathetic axons are either unmyelinated or lose their myelin sheath in the vicinity of their target tissue. Following clinical observations on conscious humans, it seems quite likely that visceral afferents of the sympathetic nerves mediate all forms of discomfort and pain, whereas parasympathetic afferents secure autonomic regulatory functions. No direct data indicate which category of viscerosensory fibers are capable of transporting non-conscious impulses and what anatomical or physiological features are required to transform these signals into conscious events (see Fig. 3). I will try to circumvent this problem in Chapter 10.

The enteric afferent fibers originate from cell bodies situated in the walls of hollow viscera of the abdominal cavity: mainly in the walls of the gastrointestinal tract and related organs such as the gallbladder. Recent authors agree on the sensory character of some of these enteric cells, which may act as sensory receptors that signal modifications in the distention, pressure, motility, and secretory activities of the gut. The afferent fibers of these enteric neurons form the rich enteric nervous plexus. Some of them, however, run far beyond the boundaries of the digestive tube, intermingled with the sympathetic fibers of the mesenteric nerves. Although there is no clear anatomical evidence that these enteric fibers enter the spinal cord and thus may send signals up to the cerebrum, physiological and psychophysical data unequivocally indicate the existence of sensations and perceptive phenomena originating from the gut. Our own data, summarized in Chapter 8, support such an assumption.

Central Projections of the Viscerosensory System

Here I shall touch on the representation of the visceral afferent apparatus in the central nervous system merely limiting the discussion to the extent necessary in order to understand better the sensations and cognitive phenomena occurring in those structures.

Visceral afferent fibers arising from cell bodies in the dorsal root ganglia, or in the nuclei of the cranial nerves outlined above, terminate in laminae I and V of the thoracic, upper lumbar, and sacral spinal cord and also in the nucleus tractus solitarius of the medulla. It must be emphasized that these visceral fibers do not have direct connections with lamina II, i.e., with the substantia

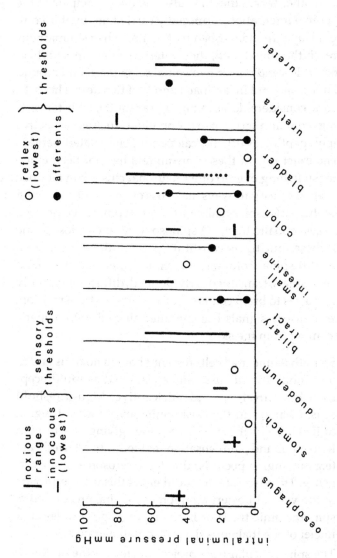

Figure 3. Thresholds of visceral afferents originating from internal organs, compiled from a large array of relevant publications by Jänig and Morrison (1986). Reprinted with kind permission of Elsevier Science - NL.

gelatinosa, in other words their impulses do not participate in the process of spinal integration supposedly carried out by this compact neuronal layer first described by Roland. When sympathetic afferents reach the spinal cord, they enter Lissauer's tract where they ascend or descend one or two spinal segments, bend around the dorsal horn, and end in laminae I and V of this dorsal horn. In addition to a considerable amount of transmitter substance P, these endings contain a series of neuropeptides, such as vasoactive intestinal polypeptide (VIP) and calcitonin gene-related peptide (CGRP). The exact role of these transmitters has not been elucidated. After switching over to other neuronal clusters in laminae I and V, viscerosensory pathways make use of one of the following four afferent tracts: (1) spinothalamic tract, (2) spinoreticular tract, (3) spinomesencephalic tract, (4) spinosolitary tract. Most of the bundles of these four tracts constitute parts of the anterolateral (extralemniscal) spinal columns, which, together with temperature and pain signals, transmit poorly-defined, diffuse, and poorly localized impulses to brain centers. In the course of transmission, these viscerosensory signals become intermingled with somatic messages coming from the skin.

1. Spinothalamic tract cells respond both to noxious and to innocuous stimuli and can be classified as multireceptive, low-threshold and nociceptive, high-threshold cells. Changes in the cardiopulmonary visceral region utilize both of these cell categories giving rise to both innocuous and pain sensations as well as to referred pain (e.g., in angina pectoris) due to viscerosomatic convergence. The visceral afferent fibers of this tract terminate in the ventral posterior region of the thalamus (medial spinothalamic tract) or in the medial and intralaminar nuclei of the thalamus (lateral spinothalamic tract).

2. The spinoreticular tract projects mainly to the midbrain tegmentum, a segment of the medial reticular formation,

and to the raphe nuclei. These medial reticular structures project farther to the intralaminar nuclei of the thalamus, which are considered to be segments of the nonspecific thalamic reticular formation. Electrophysiological and clinical observations indicate that these spinoreticular pathways carry both noxious and innocuous impulses. Among the latter are premature ventricular contractions, considered at present perhaps the only "pure" viscerosensory signals coming from the heart, which are conscious (i.e., verbally reportable; see also Chapter 8). Among painful impact somatovisceral integration is worth emphasizing, e.g., motor and skin reactions in response to cardiac pain.

3. The spinomesencephalic tract leads to definite central neuronal clusters of the midbrain, such as the parabrachial nucleus and the periaqueductal gray substance. From here innocuous and noxious messages are transmitted to the ventral posterior lateral nucleus and to the central gray matter of the thalamus. Apparently this tract may play a complementary role in the integration of viscerosomatic interaction.

4. The spinosolitary tract represents the fourth main spinal visceral afferent pathway carrying information both from large areas of internal organs and also from the skin and muscles. Thus, it can be considered as a suitable channel for viscerosomatic and viscerovisceral interactions. It originates from laminae I and V of the thoracic and sacral spinal gray and terminates on caudal neurons of the nucleus tractus solitarius. In addition to these four main tracts, the viscerosensory role of additional afferent channels cannot be excluded. For example, evidence points to the possible visceral message transmission of the spinohypothalamic tract, taking into consideration

the central role of the different nuclei of the hypothalamus in viscero- and somatosensory integration.

In surveying the data on primary visceral afferent neurons, on the spinal, medullary, mesencephalic, and thalamic projections of the viscerosensory apparatus outlined briefly above, it can be stated that most of the anatomical, electrophysiological, and neurochemical findings have been obtained in the last two decades. Thirty years ago, in completing my first monograph (Ádám, 1967), details about the aforementioned mechanisms were for the most part unknown. Our basic knowledge on cerebral cortical and cerebellar representations, however, has not changed substantially in the last quarter of a century. (Fig. 4). Only 7 years after the publication of my book, Newman (1974) had published *Visceral Afferent Functions of the Nervous System*, an outstanding monograph that analyzed in detail practically all brain structures that may play a role in viscerosensitivity. This unique work has not been surpassed to this day. This is not meant to suggest that neurophysiological research on this topic came to a standstill; on the contrary, abundant data have steadily reinforced our previous knowledge on central projections. It will suffice to mention the excellent issue of *Biological Psychology* (42, 1996) edited by Vaitl (1996), or the important volume *From the Heart to the Brain*, edited by Vaitl and Schandry (1995), or *Visceral Sensation*, edited by Cervero and Morrison (1986). These outstanding collections, however, did not alter considerably the general opinions of research workers in the field about the existence of cortical projections in the sensorimotor or in the limbic structures and about their determinant role in processing arriving visceral information. It is no wonder that Schandry and Montoya (1996) in their paper describing event-related potentials (ERPs) linked to heartbeats, emphasize the topographical role of frontal areas, the classical cortical field first explored by Danilewsky (1875) and subsequently confirmed by many authors as the site of viscerosensory signal proc-

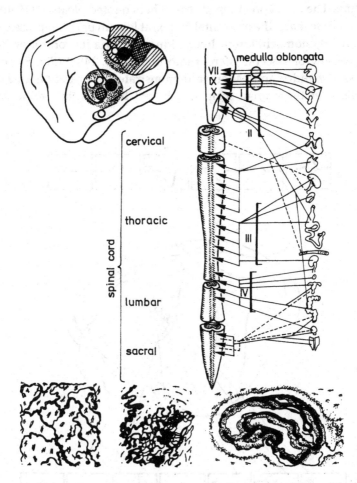

Figure 4. Schematic representation of different histological appearances of viscero-ceptors (bottom), and of visceroceptive pathways to the spinal cord and to the medulla which constitute four main tracts (I to IV, middle). The Roman numerals in the medulla refer to the appropriate cranial nerves. Top: the main cortical representations in the cat (in black, white and hatched) and the two most impor-tant primary projection areas (stripped).From Ádám (1980).

essing. The above-mentioned researchers quoted Neafsey (1990), who wrote that: "the prefrontal cortex, at least in part... represents the heart, stomach, lungs, liver, kidney, etc. via its control or its processing of visceral afferent information (p. 148)" (Fig. 5). Indeed, Schandry and Montoya demonstrated clear-cut heartbeat ERPs over the human scalp and linked them to the premotor,

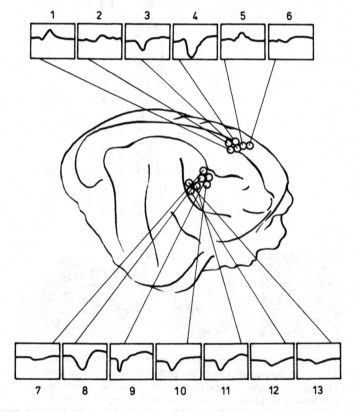

Figure 5. Scheme representing points of maximal amplitude of evoked potentials on the cat's right cortical surface to electrical stimulation of the left renal pelvis. From Ádám (1967).

orbital, and insular areas of the frontal cortex. The authors under-lined that these visceral ERPs can be deeply influenced by atten-tion and motivation, an important observation that will be discussed later (Chapter 9) and points to the possible role of limbic structures in processing visceral information, a presumption raised by us many years ago (Ádám, 1967, pp. 68–75) and rein-forced many times since. In conclusion, it can be stated that the rather simple description and scheme published 30 years ago about the central representation of viscerosensory pathways in the work just quoted, is still valid. In view of the rich recent literature on the relation between visceroception and emotion (Chapter 9) and on the rebirth of the Jamesian theory of emotion, it seems quite obvious that the earlier findings on some subcortical structures of the limbic system, including thalamic nuclei (see p. 113) as vis-cerosensory representations, are valid too.

PART *III*

Visceral Sensation and Perception

CHAPTER 7

Psychophysics of Visceral Perception in Humans

Looking back on the theoretical considerations of this essay, it seems as though the claim to quantification would be the basic criterion of the acceptance of visceral afferent events among the validated special sensory phenomena, such as olfactory, visual, and auditive processes. To be sure, the psychology of special senses is deeply intermingled with phenomena of perceiving the learned pseudoreality, i.e., of detecting and identifying the well-known illusions and even hallucinations! Also, human subjects are unable to escape the influence of these mistaken perceptions. At the same time, however, the physiology and psychology of sensations and perceptions are subject to powerful and reliable tools that can separate misperceptions from true ones. Chief among these are the law of Fechner (1860/1966) and the signal detection approach (Swets, 1964). We have undertaken some trials seeking to strip away the subjective beliefs and socially learned symptom reports (see p. 161) from the objectively quantifiable percepts. It is our view that visceroception must fulfill the same criteria as, e.g., haptic sensitivity. In other words, viscerosensory functions must be subject to the laws of psychophysics, e.g., to the basic principle of

Fechner (1860), namely $\Psi = k \cdot \log \Phi$, in which both the internal experience Ψ and the physical stimulus Φ should be measurable. It is essential to mention here that instead of the logarithmic relations originally proposed by Fechner, nowadays we apply the power function proposed by Stevens (1975): $\Psi = k \cdot \Phi^{\alpha}$, in which the exponent α depends on the modality of the Φ stimulus applied. Quantification of the internal stimulus Φ applied seems to be in most experimental and clinical cases less problematic, but the measurability of Ψ meets with several difficulties. Naturally the main obstacle is the lack of detectability of most visceral stimuli, which elicit nonreportable, unconscious behavioral or electro-physiological changes. The quantification possibilities and approaches of both components of the Fechner–Stevens principle are considered next.

Measuring the Magnitude of the Visceral Stimulus (Φ)

The solution of the exact measurement of the visceroceptive intervention is nowadays still a somewhat complicated, although not impossible task. The main reason for this situation is the difficulty in reaching visceroceptive fields situated inside the body, well under the cutaneous layers. Neither of the two main approaches seems to satisfy completely the claim of (1) exact dosing of the mechanical, chemical, electrical, or other modality of stimulus and (2) precisely achieving a purely visceroceptive (and not "contaminated" viscerosomatic) stimulation. I shall return to the problem of the difficulty of "pure" visceroception later. The two techniques applied so far in all viscerosensory experiments include either an "invasive" or a "noninvasive" approach or both.

1. The "invasive" or experimentalist approach was initiated at the beginning of this century by researchers in the Russian Pavlovian laboratories. The preliminary condition of such interventions penetrating into the lu-

mina of hollow viscera was the preparation of a great variety of chronic fistulae, like the Pavlovian pouch of the stomach, the Thiry-Vella intestinal loop, or the fistula of the ureter. These sophisticated surgical interventions, proposed originally by German physiologists, had the advantage of retaining completely intact sections of hollow organs accessible for stimulation. The artificial orifices enabled researchers and even clinical physiologists to insert different stimulating devices, such as inflatable balloons, open-ended catheters, or electrodes, into the lumina of the viscera for the purpose of achieving pneumatic or electrical stimulations, irrigation of the inner walls of the hollow organs with various solutions, and so forth. Most of these manipulations failed to produce clear-cut visceroceptive irritations; for anatomical reasons, they affected inevitably in addition to visceroceptors of the mucous membranes nonvisceroceptive structures, such as nociceptors or Pacinian-corpuscles of the serous sheets, stretch receptors of smooth muscles, and others. Looking at our own experiments conducted many years ago, carried out on humans and other animals, we were able to fulfill the requirements of a "noncontaminated," pure visceroceptive stimulation only exceptionally (dilatation of the carotid sinus by balloon in dogs; see Ádám, 1967). The bulk of our stimulation techniques was and still is a sober compromise in which we tend to exclude, more-or-less successfully, the disturbing interference of exteroceptive components when recording the effects of visceroceptive stimuli. Our "invasive" techniques in animals included the dilatation of inflatable rubber balloons in the different sections of the small and large intestines of dogs, monkeys, cats, and rats; the dilatation of the renal pelvis by the rhythmic injection of sterile solutions with the aid of ureteral catheters inserted into the orifices of ureteral fistulae of dogs; and the stretching of the carotid wall in dogs by means of small rubber balloons. In humans, duodenal Miller-Abbott- and Barthelheimer-type simple- and double-balloon catheters were inserted orally into the small intestine under X-ray control and inflated by means of a pneumatic system. All of these techniques were described in detail in Ádám (1967). Recently, human large and small intestines have been dilated by means of rubber balloons inserted into the artificial orifices of the stomata in colostomy and ileostomy patients (Ádám, Balázs, Vidos, & Keszler, 1990; Fent et al., 1998; see p. 84, 99). Unfortunately the literature on this topic does not have much in the way of better results in sine-qua-non visceral stimulation methods than ours.

2. The "noninvasive" or nonexperimentalist approach, namely, taking naturally occurring visceral functional changes into account instead of operating with artificial stimulation techniques outlined above, is in every respect more physiological than the "invasive" approach. By making use of regularly occurring compulsory functional fluctuations, such as heartbeats or intestinal contractions, and by measuring the central nervous effects of the impulses elicited by these periodic undulations, e.g., their detectability and discriminability, we may avoid many troubles and inconveniences created by "invasive" techniques. On the other side the experimenter is unable to keep under constant control or to modify according to requirements the naturally emerging periodic changes. Furthermore, these natural, regular stimuli may be too weak, to be quantified. In addition, in applying these physiological stimuli, the experimenter must be aware of the inherently double—viscero- and exteroceptive—sources, in other words, the mixed, so-

matovisceral nature of the given signals. Not to be forgotten are the dim and uncertain "symptom reports" (see the Preface). The detection of physical symptoms is always the common result of naturally occurring visceral and somatic signals mixed with previously stored, memorized information, illusions, and visceral hallucinations. In other words, they are intermingled with beliefs of the subjects about their actual internal state and ongoing real, or imagined, changes.

Taking into consideration the rather complicated and narrow conditions of quantifying the visceral stimuli (Φ) in an attempt to apply the Fechner–Stevens law, the researcher must have a modest attitude and must accept the many-sided compromises touched on above. The Latin quotation *navigare necesse est* ("it is necessary to sail") reminds us of the obligation to keep up with the times in research, to make efforts even under difficult experimental circumstances. In 1974 at a symposium of the World Congress of Physiology in New Delhi, I formulated in my lecture the demand on some psychophysics of visceroception. I had underlined the difficulties and pitfalls of such a claim, which seems to be timely even today in both measuring Φ and quantifying the Ψ value (Ádám, 1974).

Measuring the Intensity of the Visceral Experience (Ψ)

In experimental psychology, the "feeling" experienced by the subject during a psychophysical test session by means of paying forced attention directly to the internal change and reporting verbally this sensation or by manipulating some scaling device, can be substituted using different indirect methods. In the long history of our research team, with the aim of applying the Fechner–Stevens law in the field of visceral sensations, we adapted at least four experimental approaches for the quantification of Ψ. The immediate approximation of the internal "feeling" was merely one of this quadruplet of trials. The other three tests applied by us were constituents of the rich array of substitution methods capable of throwing some light on some still nebulous "feelings," usually explored merely by "introspection."

1. Recording Electrical Changes in the Brain

Since the advent of detailed research on visceral afferent processes, the electrophysiological changes following visceroceptive interventions have been thoroughly studied at almost all levels of the central nervous system. The early studies have been reviewed and summarized in several monographs (e.g., Chernigovski, 1960; Ádám, 1967; Newman, 1974). All of the results, up to the present time, proved that investigation of the alterations both of the spontaneous electroencephalographic (EEG) recordings and of ERPs is apt to elucidate several crucial brain phenomena related to the viscerosensory input. First, they proved to be appropriate tools for the elucidation of the topography of viscerosensory projection areas of the brain. Further, they proved to be suitable for the clarification of some psychophysiological functions such as sleep–wakefulness cycles, attention and arousal following viscerosensory input, and others. But, unlike electrical discharges of the peripheral afferent nerves, neither EEG nor ERP changes were appropriate for approximating the quantitative aspects of the sensory messages. Many substantial findings (see Mountcastle, 1980) demonstrate unequivocally that the frequency of impulses in a peripheral nerve fiber or bundle is directly proportional to the sensory experience of humans and other animals. This finding is the starting point of the study of the Fechner–Stevens principle in animals, where ψ represents the spike frequency instead of the intensity of "feelings" or of the sensory experience. Central EEG or ERP alterations, however, do not reflect such quantitative correlations, consequently, these changes are not utilizable in defining ψ. As far as peripheral visceral afferents are concerned, there have been no studies in humans or in other animals, on the relationship between the frequency of nerve impulses and the intensity of visceroceptive stimuli applied. The reason relates to serious technical difficulties. In animal experiments, the correlation of the impulse frequencies with the intensities of internal "feelings" cannot be studied, since in subhuman species, verbal or metaverbal reports are unthinkable. Human verification of the same correlation, on the other hand, raises major methodological uneasiness, since the recording of visceral afferent impulses *in vivo* meets serious obstacles: Viscerosensory nerve bundles run fairly deep subcutaneously, and thus cannot be easily reached by percutaneous electrodes pierced through the skin. Consequently, even though theoretically fully possible, the reliable recording of spike frequencies in human visceral afferents by applying the percutaneous human recording techniques initiated by Valbo, and Johanson (1984) has remained up to now only a chance, albeit a promising one. Thus, the approximation and validation of ψ via peripheral impulse frequencies of viscerosensory nerves and its application in the Fechner–Stevens law is nowadays impending, just as I wrote more than 20 years ago: "The combination of electrophysiological and behavioural techniques however seems to be promising in revealing the relation between the physical characteristics of visceral stimuli and the central events elicited by them" (Ádám, 1974, p. 105). It follows that other substitution techniques for obtaining ψ must be examined in order to apply this value in the Fechner–Stevens law.

2. Application of the Békésy–Blough Approximation Method

An ingeniously simple and witty circumvention of the need for quantification of the internal personal experience ψ was proposed by Hölzl *et al.* (1994) in their studies on measuring the detection of intestinal distention in human subjects. They made use of the operant discrimination test for animals created by Blough (1961) utilizing an earlier human audiometric procedure invented by Békésy (1947). In describing Békésy's witty method, Blough wrote:

> His subject listened to a soft, continuous tone and kept a telegraph key pressed down as long as he heard it. While the key was down it completed a circuit that gradually decreased the intensity of the tone. When the tone was no longer audible and the subject released the key, the tone automatically grew louder until it was heard again—whereupon the subject pressed the key, the tone faded and so on. The pen of a recorder, tracing out the fluctuations in intensity, "tracked" the subject's sensitivity on a moving piece of graph paper. (p. 114)

Hölzl found the description of Békésy's technique in Blough's papers about color discrimination in pigeons and started to apply it right away in colon distention detection trials in humans. The procedure seems to be a promising one: Recently we used it in a psychophysiological study on irritable bowel syndrom (IBS) patients (Fent et al., 1998). The subjects had to press a button if they detected a minimal "feeling" of pressure or discomfort in the abdomen. The distention volumes were automatically adjusted by the program of the computer after each button-pressing by applying a special mathematical rule in such a way that these volumes should fluctuate between the approximated sub- and suprathreshold values in order to enable the statistical computation of the distention threshold itself. Although the above approximation relies on each subjects's personal judgment about internal "feelings," the sophisticated and carefully thought-out computer program seems to render some objectivity and reliability to the procedure.

3. Application of the Signal Detection (Forced Choice) Approach

Researchers in the field of viscerosensory functions are aware that (1) internal stimuli under the conscious (reportable) threshold may elicit several nonconscious (nonreportable) responses, such as motor, autonomic, electrophysiological, and other reactions, and (2) the threshold level of consciousness (reportability) constantly fluctuates. This steady undulation of the threshold of stimulus detectability is one of the theoretical bases of the signal detection theory (Swets, 1964; Green & Swets, 1966). Although the proposers of the theory did not take into account the visceroceptive areas, we have long held the opinion that the activity of the viscerosensory system may be ranked among the characteristic models of the fluctuations of stimulus thresholds, thus "ideal" targets for the demonstration of the validity of the signal detection principle. We applied the forced choice (FC) signal detection approach repeatedly in our human viscerosensory studies (e.g., Ádám et al., 1990) and our German colleagues—independently of us—did the same (Hölzl et al., 1994, 1996). Subsequently, we have also used FC techniques in joint German–Hungarian experiments (Fent et al., 1998). Some researchers in the viscerosensory field regard signal detection and FC as separate entities (e.g., Whitehead, 1983). However, we rank FC among the varieties of signal detection approaches. The reasons for such a classification point far beyond the scope of this book.

Practical implementation of the technique requires marked warning stimuli preceding the onset or the absence of the real target stimuli to be studied (Fig. 6). The subject (the "observer" in the principle's terms) either gives a "yes" answer if the target stimulus had actually followed the warning one ("hit"), or gives the same affirmative answer if the warning stimulus was not followed by any target stimulus ("false alarm"). The alternative possibility for the subject after the warning stimulus consists of giving a "no" answer to the actually missing stimulus ("correct rejection") or giving a negative answer to a stimulus actually applied ("missed"). After a rather considerable amount of randomly applied and not applied stimuli preceded always by warning signals, the experimenter will be able to compute the signal to

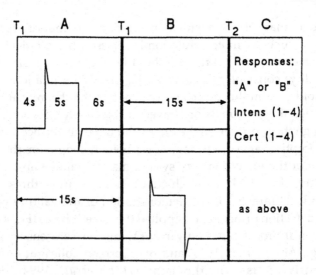

Figure 6. Diagram of a forced-choice trial. T_1 and T_2 are warning tones, A and B are observation intervals, C is the response interval for ratings in four points about intensity ("intens") and certainty ("cert") judgments. Reprinted from Hölzl *et al.* (1996) with kind permission of Elsevier Science - NL.

noise ratio of the subject's replies, as well as to construct the "receiver's operating characteristic" (ROC) curves of the subject (the "receiver"), considered to represent not only the threshold conditions, but also some other personality traits of the subject (e.g., sensation-seeking, success orientation). Of course we are mainly interested in the degree of reliability of the FC approach in quantifying a given viscerosensory Ψ value. According to our conjectures, FC techniques may tackle the "real" visceral experience more faithfully than the Békésy–Blough approach, since the latter assumes some kind of preconscious or nonconscious sensation to be detected by external pressure, namely, by the warning stimulus triggering forced attention to this nonconscious sensory event. But the FC approaches still remain indirect approximations, and I am not in the least optimistic that more exact and reliable methods in quantitatively defining the visceral Ψ value can be discovered. This rather skeptical view was reinforced by a fourth, this time straightforward and direct approach to approximate the visceral Ψ value.

4. "Direct" Approximation of the Validity of the Fechner-Stevens Law

After the above short description of the three substitution methods for estimating the magnitude of Ψ, I now turn to the treatment of the immediate determination of the internal experience evoked by visceral stimulation mentioned in the first paragraph of this chapter. Of course, in the early history of psychophysics, "substitution" approaches could not be considered, since their fundamental principles, e.g., the above-treated Fechner law, were based on evidently suprathreshold, conscious (reportable) environmental Φ stimuli, such as visual, auditive, tactile, and the like. It is no wonder that after the advent of viscerosensory research tendencies, the demand for a visceral direct psychophysical quantification appeared in the literature, although it was obvious from the very beginning of this claim that the "direct" estimation of any kind of stimulus, even of the thoroughly studied visual or auditive one, is after all an "indirect" approximation. The verbal report or the manipulation of any kind of scaling device (e.g., of the Békésy techniques) does not throw light on the very nature of the sensation (Ψ) itself, consequently the real "direct" measurement of the magnitude of any sensation—including the visceral one—remains an unsolved problem. In this respect, every sensory modality, including viscerosensory signals, can be judged by the same standard, the only line of demarcation—although a stressed one—being the high threshold of detection (reportability) of the visceral input in comparison with external stimuli.

Taking notice of the above rather evident and crucial circumstance, I will briefly expound on a pilot trial for the formulation of the Fechner–Stevens law concerning visceroception and the pitfalls of this attempt. A group of male colostomy patients were examined in three consecutive experimental sessions each. A rubber balloon was inserted into the colonic stoma orifice applying the usual technique described by us earlier (Ádám *et al.*, 1990; Fent *et al.*, 1998). The catheter of the balloon was connected to a special mechanical pump system driven by a computer. After identification of the minimal detectable (reportable) threshold by asking the subject to push a button when some minimal, dim feeling of tension, pressure, or discomfort was observed, we started a Békésy-type ascending and descending scaling (Békésy, 1947). This method, also called the *method of limits,* consists of estimating the detection threshold by progressively increasing the intensity of the stimulus until the subject reports that he or she perceives it, or by progressively decreasing the intensity until the subject reports being unable to perceive it. The subject was instructed to follow and to estimate the "feelings" to the gradual inflation and deflation of the balloon by manipulating a visual analogue scale (VAS). The VAS consisted of a sliding potentiometer, the tuning from 0 to 10 being visualized on the screen of a monitor placed 1 meter in front of the prone subject and with the sliding plastic potentiometer within reach.

Our results seem to reinforce the validity of the Fechner–Stevens power law in the field of the visceromechanical modality. The linear relationship between the volume of air in the inflated balloon and the estimated "feeling" of distention displayed on the VAS is evident on a semi logarithmic scale, whereas a double logarithmic plot shows a somewhat bent line (Fig. 7). The latter relationship needs further analysis, but the statement of Stevens (1979) cannot be denied:

> the psychophysical power law now stands as the most pervasive and perhaps the best-supported quantitative generalization in psychology. There appears to be no exception to the rule that on all prothetic continua the subjective magnitude Ψ grows as the stimulus magni-

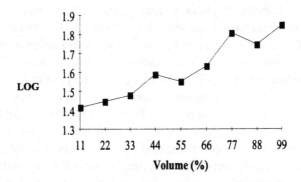

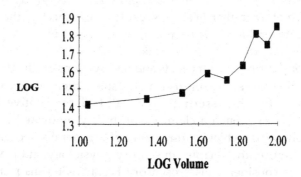

Figure 7. Diagram of grand average representations of the results of nine experimental sessions displaying the Ψ values of the Fechner–Stevens law (in log scale, see text) to different distention volumes of the large intestine expressed in volume % (top) and in log volume (bottom).

tude Φ raised to a power. Hence the formula may be written $\Psi = K\Phi^{\alpha}$ where α is the exponent. Conveniently, in double logarithmic coordinates, this equation becomes a line whose slope corresponds to the exponent. (p. 868)

All four approaches to the approximation of the Ψ value, namely, the latter "direct" estimation and the former (recording electrical changes, the Békésy–Blough method, the signal detection approach) trials, apparently have common drawbacks, since it is well known that all perceptual decisions are influenced by a series of nonperceptual factors called *response bias*. Most of these response bias components are in fact personality traits. For example, some subjects are success-oriented and tend to give affirmative answers even when they are hesitant, since both a hit and a false alarm reinforce their motivational attitudes. Other subjects tend to have a reserved attitude, they respond positively only if they are absolutely certain about detection since they want to have a conservative personal image. Unfounded boasting and endless, groundless hesitation are always present as extreme behavioral patterns of response bias in a randomly recruited group of subjects. The other, rather health-psychological, aspect of the same personality problem has been amply discussed in works about symptom reporters (e.g., Pennebaker, 1982).

Considering all of the facts and observations outlined in this chapter, there are seen to be insurmountable difficulties in creating conditions for the assertion of a valid visceroceptive Fechner–Stevens law. Such a claim is still highly motivated and remains one of the chief requirements of a generally recognized, solid visceroceptive chapter in sensory physiology and psychology. If we consider a viscerosensory Fechner–Stevens principle merely a conjecture (evidently an overstatement), we may add with good reason that conjectures play an important stimulating role not only in mathematics, but in other scientific disciplines as well.

CHAPTER *8*

Visceral Perception through Learning

In the foregoing chapters on the psychophysics of viscerosensory stimuli, we were dealing exclusively with "inherent" visceroceptive events, i.e., phenomena actually occurring in the "real time" of our experimental situations and our observations. In other words, we could not and did not pay attention to the past of these internal changes, and we did not know anything about the ontogenetic history of the viscerosensory events studied in our subjects. That is why quotes appeared around the term *feelings*; however, it would be proper to name these reportable viscerosensory phenomena "*inherent*" in visceral sensations or perceptions. It has been our presumption for many years that in adults, these inherent conscious phenomena are the resultants of long and complex learning processes in which at least two main components necessarily take part, namely, (1) inborn abilities to detect, to recognize, and eventually to name viscerosensory signals and (2) reinforcing (mediating) inborn stimuli of somatic character originating from receptors from the inside or from the surface of the body (contact receptors), eventually from a given distance (telereceptors). Accidentally social reinforcing stimuli may have a role in creating "inherent"

87

visceral sensitivity (e.g., bladder and rectal distention detection under the pressure of the social environment).

Inborn Visceral Sensations

Paintal (1986) enumerated five visceral reportable sensations that can be observed in any animal as innate features, namely, breathlessness, satiation of hunger, satiation of thirst, bladder fullness, and rectal fullness. The sporadic data in the available literature agree with this limited list of inborn abilities. Among those who attempted to complete this list are Kline and Bidder (1946), who described subjective sensations associated with extrasystoles. In addition to the above enumeration of innate visceral sensations, we are inclined to regard all other conscious and nonconscious viscerosensory events either as inherently "finished products" of the individual subject's life span, or as evidently learned, acquired results of explorable conditioning or cognitive processes that took place in the subject's past. The so-called "physical symptoms" so amply discussed in the recent psychophysiological literature (e.g., Leventhal, Meyer, & Nerenz, 1980; Pennebaker, 1982, 1996) cannot be taken into consideration here, since from a strict physiological standpoint they represent excessively mixed sensory phenomena from symptom reports following blood sugar changes up to feelings of different complex emotions and pain.

Scientific investigation has no tools at present to collect proofs and to furnish evidence in favor of the above-described hypothesis, especially considering that even the acquired, learned character of the meager items in Paintal's list cannot be excluded either. Our own early experiments on puppies (Moiseeva, 1952) indicated that visceroceptive conditioning is easily feasible in young dogs. Based on these and other data from the Pavlovian laboratories, we presumed long ago that visceroceptive signals predominate over external ones immediately after birth, while later, at the age of 1½ to 2 months in dogs, the relation of the two kinds of inputs is reversed: Information from the external environment becomes more significant than the visceral variety. Moiseeva also found that in the rabbit embryo in the uterus, stimuli from the visceral field may inhibit the motor responses of the fetus. All of these observations point to the possibility that in the early stages of ontogenesis, the role of visceroceptive signals is more important than that of external messages. These assumptions were amply treated in Ádám (1967, pp. 8–9) and seem to be in agreement with the relatively new hypothesis of "competition of cues" by Pennebaker (1982, 1996). This author emphasizes that if attention is directed toward signals from inside the body, then visceral perception prevails, and vice versa—if attention is drawn to external cues, exteroception inhibits visceroception. Apparently, visceral messages have an important survival value in the fetus and newborn, and consequently they triumph.

The Learning Process

Returning to Paintal's enumeration of innate conscious visceral sensations, the careful researcher gets the impression that even among those five classes of visceral signals certain processes may be the results of early learning mechanisms. Bladder and rectal fullness, i.e., the urgent need to void, are first of all "suspects" in this regard. This "suspicion" was based on our early data on visceroceptive conditioning, which created the idea that most (if not all) early reportable sensations labeled as "innate" are really the consequences of learning, all the more so because in mammals some kind of conditioning procedures start even before birth, i.e., in fetal life. That is why the term *inherent* seems to be more adequate for such early features than *innate*, as treated in the foregoing pages.

A considerable amount of the research efforts of the author and his group was devoted for a relatively long period of time to elucidation of the background mechanisms of the double-faced visceral input and, thus, solution of the dilemma: genetically inherited or individually learned?

The following pages review the main results of our investigations in light of the relevant literature in order to draw some conclusions as to the nature of visceral information processing. The original paradigm of using viscerosensory input as conditional stimuli (CS) in a classical conditioning situation had first been suggested in the Pavlovian laboratory by Bykov and Ivanova (Bykov, 1947). They applied the irrigation of the gastric mucosa as CS and the injection of water into the stomach as unconditional stimulus (US), thus producing a hyposmotic situation with subsequent diuresis. After pairing the CS and US 20–25 times, a marked diuresis could be observed even if the rinsing of the gastric mucosa was not accompanied by introduction of water. Consequently, the stimulus applied to the receptors of the stomach wall evoked a state similar to the one resulting from hyposmosis. The new paradigm was worked out in detail by Airapetyants (1952) and his co-workers, who carried out mechanical, chemical and thermal stimulation of the gastrointestinal (GI) mucosa of various topographies and in several sites of the genital tract as CS, and alimentary as well as defensive reactions as US. Airapetyants summarized his group's data in demonstrating the validity of the main laws of Pavlovian conditioning in the field of elementary learning elicited by visceral signals. This laboratory did not, however, pay attention to the characteristics of the viscerosensory phenomena themselves, and their achievements can be regarded as a series of rather extensive pilot studies on the interrelations of interoceptive and exteroceptive, i.e., viscerosensory and somatosensory conditioning, undertaken mainly on dogs.

Our own visceroceptive learning studies on dogs were based initially on the above data. Our early aim was merely to extend these Russian results to the stimulation of a typical vascular receptor area, the carotid sinus, and to a characteristic hollow organ not studied before, the renal pelvis and the ureter. Parallel to the control and eventual reinforcement of the Pavlovian data, we succeeded in extending those studies to the symmetry of renal sensory input, the compensatory mechanisms between paired viscerosensory messages, and other related areas. In addition to alimentary conditioning using food as US and visceral stimuli as CS, EEG arousal was used as US in other experiments, also on dogs, in which the CS was also the distention of the renal pelvis or of the carotid sinus (Fig. 8). These initial experimental series demonstrated unequivocally that impulses from hollow organs other than the GI tract and from the vascular system reach higher brain areas and, in addition to their regulatory role, well known from classical physiological data, might be the triggers of complex behavioral, i.e., learned, reactions. An incidental finding also proved to be significant, namely, that weak pelvic and carotid distentions may initiate arousals of the EEG and evoked potentials too. For unbiased observers from the United States and Western Europe, the findings on the discriminatory ability of the brain concerning stimuli arriving from the symmetrical kidneys, from pelvic and ureteral loci 10 cm apart, or from duodenal sites 10–30 cm apart seemed somewhat inconceivable when first published (e.g., Ádám & Mészáros, 1957; Ádám, Mészáros, & Zubor, 1957; Ádám, Mészáros, Lehotzky, & Kelemen, 1960). Later they were integrated in the framework of my early monograph (Ádám, 1967) and reinforced by data obtained using operant conditioning techniques on rhesus monkeys with isolated intestinal loops (Slucki *et al.*, 1965).

Incidentally, the discriminatory ability concerning weak signals from the intestines was demonstrated by us, in parallel to the above conditioning experiments, making use of the so-called "habituation discrimination test" both on dogs (Ádám *et al.*, 1960) and on humans (Ádám, Preisich, Kukorelli, & Kelemen, 1965). A typi-

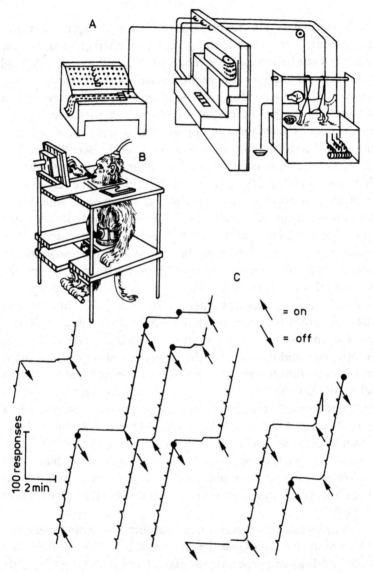

Figure 8. Setup for classical (A) and for instrumental visceroceptive conditioning (B) from the gut. (C) Cumulative curve of operant responses. Arrows indicate onset and offset of weak intestinal distention of the isolated loop. From Ádám (1980).

cal experimental session began by inserting double-balloon catheters into the duodenum and subsequently allowing both for the
human subjects and for the dogs to attain a steady resting alpha
rhythm of the EEG. In the background of this alpha state a weak,
near-threshold distention was achieved (at site A of the gut), which
evoked the desynchronization (beta activity) of the EEG. After
repeated alpha states and repeated application of the distention at
site A, habituation (lasting alpha state) could be observed. In the
background of this habituated EEG, another distention was
achieved with a second balloon (at site B of the gut) situated a
given distance (in humans, about 15 cm) from site A. Desynchronization reappeared, which meant that the brain could discriminate
between signals arriving from sites A and B of the intestines,
respectively (see Fig. 9).

The first analytical survey of these data (Ádám, 1967) threw
light on the uneasiness of our technique of visceral stimulation,

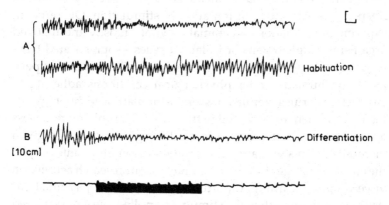

Figure 9. Plot of a habituation discrimination test on the dog. After habituation of
the desynchronization following distention of the gut at site A, a new distention
at site B at a distance of 10 cm re-evoked a desynchronization of the EEG. Bottom
line: time calibration (in sec) and the sign of the gut stimulus (thick block). Similar
tests performed on humans yielded identical results. From Ádám (1967).

which has remained a problem up to the present. The "macromethod" we used on dogs and on humans, i.e., rhythmic distention of the visceral wall, was "not delicate and accurate enough to be used to establish some particular properties of the end-organs" (p. 22). This statement, formulated more than 30 years ago, turned out to reveal a crucial, still unsolved, drawback of all *in vivo* visceral sensitivity studies: the lack of adequate, precise stimulation techniques in experimentation on humans and other animals. This means that neither mechanical (distention by balloon or irrigation of the mucous membrane), nor electrical (monopolar or bipolar, sine curve or square wave), nor chemical (acidic, basic, or neutral), nor thermal (warm or cold) stimulation can avoid the involvement of somatic end organs in the minute changes elicited by such a stimulation, even if it was aimed exclusively at visceral mechano-, chemo-, or thermoreceptors of the mucosa or of the smooth muscular layers of the walls. *In vivo* neurophysiological technology had and still has no reliable and precise methods to bypass somatic endings, especially free nerve fibers, i.e., nociceptors, at initiation of stimulation. Of course in experimental situations on animals—whole, mostly anesthetized organisms, single organs or isolated tissues—sophisticated techniques are already and will be even more available, but in experiments on humans under physiological conditions adhering to strict ethical rules, refined visceral stimulation technology remains a problem to be solved in the future. The only more-or-less appropriate and reliable tool in modifying the effect of a given visceral stimulus was and still is the variation of the intensity of the stimulating agent. At the beginning of our research activity on visceroceptive learning, unfortunately we did not pay much attention to the strength of the stimuli we applied; we were satisfied merely to restrict ourselves not to provoke pain—judging from behavioral reactions of the animal or verbal reports of the human subject. Frankly, this practice was an erroneous imitation of the Pavlovian routine. Later, in both animal and human experimentation dealing with visceroceptive influence on behavior, the intensity aspect of the stimulus was always carefully under control as described in the previous chapter on human psychophysics.

The first striking urge to take into consideration the intensities of the visceral stimuli applied was the failure to repeat and reproduce our early successful finding, obtained on rhesus monkeys with chronic isolated intestinal fistulae, on the intestinal control of operant lever-pressing behavior (Slucki et $al.$, 1965). In those experiments, the presence of the rhythmic distention of the small intestine served as S^D or S^Δ, respectively. Trying to reproduce the monkey experiments this time on rats, supplied with isolated intestinal loops and visceral stimulating electrodes, we could not demonstrate that weak GI electrical or mechanical stimuli can serve as discriminative signals in a lever-pressing operant situation. The failure could be transformed into success when applying more intensive—rather aversive than pain-producing—stimuli. Bárdos and Ádám had undertaken a kind of behavioral calibration of GI stimuli too (Bárdos & Ádám, 1978, 1980; Bárdos, Nagy, & Ádám, 1980). The presumption was increasingly confirmed that the intervention of some somatic receptor structures in the process of irritation following mechanical or electrical gut stimuli could be the cause of the "breakthrough" of subthreshold stimulation to become suprathreshold in controlling operant responding. Apparently in the early operant conditioning experiments on monkeys, "contaminated" visceral impulses, i.e., mixed viscerosomatic suprathreshold signals, reached the appropriate brain centers evoking the initiation and the cessation of operant behavior after alimentary reinforcements (Slucki et $al.$, 1965) (Fig. 8C).

In all probability, such "contaminated" viscerosomatic impulses served as CS in some of our early human conditioning studies in which we did not pay any special attention to the strength of the visceral stimulation provided they reached the EEG threshold of evoking the blocking of the alpha waves and the onset of beta activity. In two different series of experiments, beta activity had been initiated in two groups of resting human subjects, namely, by weak duodenal balloon distention (Ádám *et al.*, 1965) in one group, and by weak electrical stimulation of the neck of the uterus in the other group (see Kukorelli, Ádám, Gimes, & Tóth, 1972). These internal stimuli happened to be very moderate, since the subjects did not report any sensations of pressure, shock, or discomfort at the moment of marked EEG desynchronization. Subsequently, by reinforcing verbally ("attention: you feel now the pressure or shock") those nonreportable duodenal or uterine stimuli, the visceral signals of nonconscious intensity became detectable: The subjects reported their subjective feelings by pressing the appropriate button. In this way the "subjective threshold" (detection of the internal stimulus) and the "objective threshold" (triggering beta waves on the EEG) became close or identical to each other. We could construct in both experiments typical "curves of perception" or "slopes of becoming conscious" (Fig. 10), which proved to be crucial illustrative tools in our later concept about the double character, the borderline nature of the viscerosensory system (Ádám, 1983; see also Chapter 10 of this book).

The two main issues outlined in this chapter, namely, the share of the somatosensory influence in viscerosensory conditioning and the inherent versus learned character of visceral sensations and perceptions, seem to constitute the cutting edge of the whole visceroception problem. That is why we showed and still show great concern about these two questions. Consequently, we tried to tackle the problems in a specially designed experimental series undertaken on 22 male colostomy patients (Ádám *et al.*, 1990). The sygmoid colon of each subject was distended using a rubber balloon inserted about 10 cm into the colon through the artificial stoma in three sessions spanning 3 weeks. Each session included several signal-detection and learning tasks. During each task, the patient received the colon stimulus (the "signal") 25 times randomly paired with masking auditory or annular skin pressure stimuli (administered through pneumatic rubber tires around the

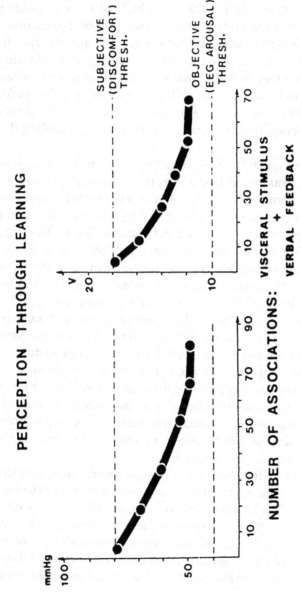

Figure 10. Visceral perception diagrams of duodenal and uterine stimulations. Similar curves of "becoming conscious" (thick lines) can be obtained by associating gut (pneumatic, left) or uterine (electrical, right) stimulation with verbal stimuli. Note that the subjective threshold of mild discomfort (upper broken line) will approach the objective threshold of EEG arousal (lower broken line).From Ádám, (1983).

stoma or 15 cm medial to it on the abdominal wall). These masking (warning) stimuli were administered in series of 50, representing the "noise" in signal-detection paradigms. The subjects had to indicate after each administration of the warning noise stimulus whether or not they believed that the colon stimulus had been presented simultaneously. In all three sessions, learning tasks were included using musical reinforcement of successful detection trials through the computer conducting and controlling the session.

The experimental procedure yielded data that could answer some of the questions outlined above, thus reinforcing our earlier results: (1) inherent sensitivity to colon distention could be proven in 16 of 22 patients even before conditioning trials; (2) subsequent auditive reinforcement improved detection ability by learning, thus converting nonconscious visceral input into conscious perception via operant training (Fig. 11); (3) the warning (at the same time as "noise") stimuli made colon distention detection more difficult, because they had a masking effect. This masking influence was less marked, when auditory warning was applied, than annular skin pressure applied 15 cm from the stoma orifice, and the latter effect was less explicit than skin pressure applied directly around the artificial orifice. To summarize, the results obtained on these 22 patients seem to point to the inherently mixed nature of colon impulses. The contribution of external stimuli, such as somatic interstitial, peritoneal, and dermal signals, seems probable. Instrumental learning trials were again effective in significantly improving gut distention perception.

Summing up the above series of experiments, some subjects can detect gut distention and show an improvement in detection with training. This finding is in accordance with our early data (Ádám et al., 1965) on human duodenal sensitivity, and with subsequent findings on the mechanoreceptive conscious phenomena originating from different sections of the GI tract (see Whitehead, 1983, and Appendix II of this book). The morphological

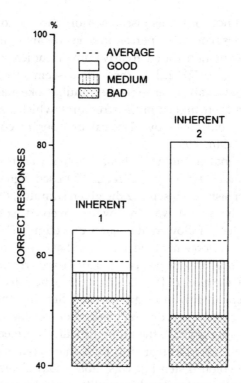

Figure 11. Correct responses to threshold intestinal distentions in a group of 22 subjects (good, medium, and bad perceivers) before (inherent 1) and after (inherent 2) learning. Reprinted from Ádám et al. (1990) with the permission of Cambridge University Press.

background of such innocuous and noxious sensations has been sufficiently elucidated and summarized by Jänig and Morrison (1986). Because 16 of the 22 subjects investigated revealed a tendency for colon distention detection even prior to learning trials, inherent sensitivity can be hypothesized. Subsequent training using an operant conditioning procedure (reinforcement schedule) improved detection ability at least in the good perceivers. The conversion of nonconscious viscerosensory input into reportable and more-or-less conscious perception via operant training procedures has been demonstrated in early human studies (Ádám, 1967; Kukorelli *et al.*, 1972). All of these data seem to confirm our hypothesis that weak viscerosensory stimuli evoke mainly nonreportable events in higher brain structures which become conscious when reinforced by classical or operant conditioning procedures (Ádám, 1983).

The cardinal question is, what has actually been stimulated? It is well known that the most frequently used signal-detection procedure consists of presenting the given stimulus, the "signal," simultaneously with a warning, well perceived, stimulus, the "noise." We have followed the same procedure. This warning stimulus, as a component of the noise, also has masking properties because the simultaneous presentation of this clearly recognizable stimulus with the more or less hidden signal to be detected renders the detection procedure more difficult. It is clear that the closer the hypothetical central nervous representations of the two stimuli (the noise and the signal), the more difficult the detection of the latter becomes. It is not surprising, then, that in our experimental situation the colon distention was more easily detected by the patients when it was masked by auditory masking stimuli than when it was presented simultaneously with abdominal annular pressure. In addition, the two different topographical locations of the abdominal skin stimuli, namely, around the stoma (proximal skin) or 15 cm medial to it (distant skin), allowed examination of the possibility that colon distention affected skin mechanoreceptors too. If the proximal skin pressure exerts a more explicit masking effect on colon distention detection than the distant skin stimulus, then discrimination of overlapping stimuli (i.e., colon+proximal skin) is a more difficult task for the subjects than discrimination of the less overlapping stimuli (i.e., colon+distant skin). This was confirmed in the second session of the series described above. It must be emphasized, however, that both skin stimuli were applied to the same dermatome (Th 9 or 10) of the given subject, so the possible contribution of dermal, peritoneal, and interstitial receptors to the detection of the distention of the bowel cannot be excluded.

In most of our earlier visceroceptive studies (see Ádám, 1967), the surface of the hollow organs stimulated had been rinsed with anesthetizing fluid in order to prove that local anesthesia blocks the viscerosensory effect, i.e., that true visceral input has been studied. Following this routine, it was decided to rinse the colon at the end of the last session with saline and subsequently with Novocain-like anesthetizing fluid (lidocaine 10%). Interestingly enough, neither the saline nor the anesthetic abolished gut distention detection. The most plausible explanation of this finding must rely on the anatomical localization of distention-sensitive mechanoreceptors of the colon, which are seemingly situated in the muscular layer of the bowel. The application of saline or a small amount of Novocain-like fluid could be attention-enhancing instead of abolishing the gut-detection ability of the subjects. However, two other explanations may be considered: first, the "time effect" of the training, because the anesthetizing fluid was presented at the end of the three-session series, and second, the irrigation effect of the fluid, which cleansed the mucosa and thus improved the accessibility and performance of the receptors.

In summary, the colon-distention detection experiments seem to point to the borderline nature of these viscerosensory events as far as consciousness is concerned. Signal detection and subsequent training were necessary to elicit reported sensations from the covert background of diffuse abdominal impulses. The results point furthermore to the inherently mixed nature of colon impulses: Exteroceptive "contamination," i.e., the contribution of somatic interstitial, peritoneal, and dermal receptors, cannot be excluded. The anatomical and physiological basis of colon sensations relies on the mucosal and muscular receptor apparatus summarized by Jänig and Morrison (1986). In any event, the results of this study strongly challenge the traditional widespread view in internal medicine and surgery as to the "insensibility"of visceral organs, especially the gut. They point to the existence of inherent, although foggy intestinal sensations and to the role of learning in the conscious perception of this type of sensitivity.

CHAPTER *9*

Hemispheric Lateralization of Signal Processing

In chapter 7 dealing with the viscerosensory stimulus to be applied, I discussed the "noninvasive" or nonexperimentalist approaches, which make use of periodically and naturally occurring visceral fluctuations and of the physiological visceral impulses provoked by them. Parallel to the admission of the limits and difficulties of applying "invasive" techniques in human experiments on the viscerosensory system (see pp. 76), inspired by the original approach of the Laceys (Lacey & Lacey, 1978), we started to use the very attractive and simple heartbeat detection technique. Of course we knew of the early attempts of Brener and Jones (1974) and McFarland (1975), but it was Whitehead, Drescher, Heiman, and Blackwell (1977) who convinced us to include the heartbeat detection trials among our human viscerosensory methods. This suggestion proved to be timely, since in the early 1980s we sought "noninvasive" human experimental techniques adequate to investigate the hemispheric preference problem. Earlier we were unsuccessful in tackling the issue in rat experiments on visceroception (Ádám, Bárdos, Hoffmann, & Nagy, 1977). Jones (1994), in his important review article on this methodology, listed

103

48 published experiments in the years between 1974 and 1989 and another 54 unpublished studies (abstracts and dissertations) in that span. Thus, it was clear that this rather unsophisticated trend had become highly popular among scientists, mostly psychologists. This popularity had and still has many benefits, such as several research teams working on the same or related problems and being able to exchange ideas and experiences, to control and reproduce each other's data, and so forth. There are at the same time some disadvantages to being fashionable, such as a peculiar "blindness of criticism" (recall the overpopularized "memory transfer" trend in the late 1960s or the oversimplified "biofeedback" campaign in the 1970s). A lack of critical thinking is not foreign to some authors working in the field of heartbeat perception. Namely, the common view regards the latter as a kind of "visceral perception." However, it is clear to physiologists, experimental psychologists, and cardiologists that this is, as much a somatic and auditive sensory event (we detect heartbeats, more closely the pulses of the large arteries during systoles, through skin and interstitial receptors and even through the noise of the arterial blood flow of the organ of Corti in the inner ear) as it is a viscerosensory phenomenon (afferent nerve bundles run from the atrial and ventricular heart receptors, from the nerve endings of the great arteries of the chest through the vagus and the glossopharyngeal to the medulla transmitting mechanical events of the systole). Of course, this essential circumstance did not hinder us in our decision to study signal processing during heartbeat detection, since, as discussed (pp. 100–101), all viscerosensory functions analyzed so far dealt with mixed, visceral and somatic messages and we raised the provocative question: does "pure" viscerosensory input exist at all?

We decided in favor of the heartbeat technique because it seemed a simple noninvasive approach to examine whether, as in processing a variety of visual, tactile, and auditory information, the visceral input also is detected by the nondominant hemisphere. Almost simultaneously with the pioneering papers of Kimura (1961), Milner, Taylor, and Sperry, (1968), Mountcastle (1975), and Sperry (1977) we tried to extend these data to the viscerosensory field by hypothesizing that visceral input might be similarly processed by the nonverbal hemisphere. Our first attempt undertaken on rats, using visceroceptive conditioning and then removing one hemisphere, happened to be unsuccessful: We did not observe any significant difference in processing conditional reactions originating from the gut after hemispherectomy in comparison with the viscerosensory learning of the rats with intact brain hemispheres (Ádám et al., 1977). This failure was the very moment of decision in favor of the use of the viscerosomatic heartbeat detection technique as indicated above. We showed from the beginning of our attempts great concern about the hemispheric lateralization problem. In addition to the above-mentioned results on nonvisceral signal processing by the nondominant hemisphere, we knew of the findings of Hantas, Katkin, and Reed (1984) and Montgomery and Jones (1984) indicating that right hemisphere preferent individuals detect their heartbeats more accurately than left preferents, among right-handed subjects.

Weisz and her co-workers in our laboratory started several series in succession, applying the heartbeat detection technique suggested by Whitehead et al., (1977). Except for the first investigation, which examined the role of self-focused attention (Weisz, Balázs, & Ádám, 1988) (see p. 111), the information processing of the nondominant hemisphere was always in the forefront of our interest. The main findings were as follows:

1. Heartbeat discrimination accuracy is influenced by the direction of lateral visual fixation of the eyes, fixation to the left (right hemisphere activation) resulting in better performance than fixation to the right (left hemisphere activation). Further, hemispheric preference, deter-

mined by conjugate lateral eye movements (CLEMs), affected the ability to detect heartbeats even when subjects were gazing laterally; left-movers were always better heartbeat discriminators than right-movers (Weisz, Balázs, Láng, & Ádám, 1990) (Fig. 12).

This result might be interpreted as the consequence of the greater resting, "background" neural activity in the preferred hemisphere. Assuming that the activity increase in one hemisphere, created by lateral gaze of appropriate direction, is algebraically added to the resting activity, activation of the preferred hemisphere will result in greater total hemispheric activity than activation of the nonpreferred hemisphere. Alternatively, it is also possible that the preferred hemisphere might be activated by contralateral visual fixation to a greater extent than the nonpreferred hemisphere. EEG and cerebral blood flow studies may help to clarify this issue.

Overall, heartbeat detection performance of bidirectionals was intermediate between left-movers and right-movers, but, contrary to our expectation, lateral visual fixation did not influence their heartbeat discrimination accuracy. One possible explanation for this finding might be that bidirectional subjects are more resistant to procedures that aim to create differential hemispheric activation. This assumption could be tested by studying the effects of other types of hemispheric activation procedures, such as unilateral nostril breathing.

2. In monocular viewing conditions, due to an activational imbalance between the cerebral hemispheres, an asymmetry could be observed in heartbeat detection performance. Namely, perception was more accurate when viewing with the left eye (right hemisphere dominance),

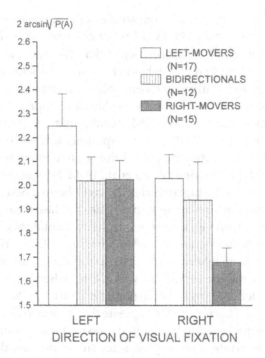

Figure 12. Correct heartbeat detections and standard errors in right hemisphere preferents (left-movers, $n=17$), left hemisphere preferents (right movers, $n=15$), and bidirectionals ($n=12$). Reprinted from Weisz *et al.* (1990) with the permission of Cambridge University Press.

the right eye being patched. Power spectral analysis of the heart period variability showed that the amount of heart rate fluctuations depends on the viewing eye. Only viewing with the left eye produced a significant increase of the midfrequency peak. Hence, left monocular viewing results in an increased sympathetic influence on the sinoatrial cardiac node (Weisz, Szilágyi, Láng, & Ádám, 1992; Weisz, Balázs, & Ádám, 1994). Additional evidence supporting the hemispheric activation effect of monocular viewing comes from studies of performance on verbal and spatial tasks (Weisz et al., 1994) as well as the accuracy of heartbeat perception (Weisz et al., 1990). Heartbeat perception has been repeatedly shown to be a predominantly right hemispheric function, and right hemispheric activation was shown to improve its accuracy (Hantas et al., 1984; Montgomery & Jones, 1984; Weisz et al., 1990). In our experiment, heartbeats were more accurately perceived during left-eye than during right-eye viewing (Weisz et al., 1990). We suggested that left-eye viewing activates the right hemisphere, which, in turn, results in an improvement of heartbeat perception. However, a right hemispheric mental rotation task was better performed when viewing with the right eye (left hemispheric activation), and the accuracy on a left hemispheric verbal task was greater when viewing with the left eye (right hemispheric activation) (Weisz et al., 1994). This result was opposite that expected. A possible interpretation for this is that task-irrelevant visual information might act as a distractor and, consequently, interfere with cognitive processing. If so, the more irrelevant visual information a hemisphere receives, the less effective it is in cognitive processing. Another explanation might be that the activational optimum for the cognitive tasks used is low. As there is an inverted-U-shaped relationship between activation and performance (Yerkes–Dodson law), monocular viewing might produce supraoptimal activation of the contralateral hemisphere. Nonetheless, these findings support the hypothesis that monocular viewing influences hemispheric functions, but the direction of performance changes cannot be explained by supposing a simple positive relationship between activation level and performance.

3. A gender difference was demonstrated in connection with eye movements and hemispheric preference. It was found that in males, eye movements evoked by bilateral visual stimulation (BVS) are related to cognitive performance. Specifically, males with a preference of leftward eye movements are relatively more accurate on a spatial than a verbal task, whereas, the opposite is true for males preferring rightward eye movements. In females, such a relationship was not observed (Weisz & Ádám, 1993). The main finding of this study—that in males, eye movements evoked by BVS are related to cognitive performance—strongly indicates that eye movements have a close relationship with hemispheric preference. The direction of the effect is in accordance with expectations, based on the results of brain stimulation, brain damage, and CLEM studies.

The other findings of this study seems to offer additional, albeit indirect, support for the hypothesis that eye movement direction during the BVS procedure reflects hemispheric preference. In males, body mass index (BMI) was found to negatively correlate with the ratio of leftward eye movements, a result similar to those found in CLEM studies. CLEM studies were interpreted as indicating a connection between hemispheric preference and obesity, left hemisphere preferent individuals being more obese than right hemisphere preferent ones. We expected that in our experiment this connection would be reflected in a relationship between eye movements and BMI. For males this expectation proved to be true, and the direction of the relationship was the same as found in CLEM studies.

The three groups of results, outlined above, in addition to some minor findings, have one common denominator of rather significant consequences: they seem to reinforce those data, that point to the lateralization of signal processing in the brain in general and of viscerosomatic heartbeat detection in particular. The findings may have two more corollaries, one related to physiological backgrounds of attention, and the other to hemispheric control of emotion.

Attention or Lifelong Conditioning?

A rather unusual, almost "bizarre" finding in the course of the initiation of the heartbeat detection approach was the "mirror effect": It was found that subjects performed heartbeat discrimination more accurately when facing a mirror. The mirror experiment was a peculiar combination of the heartbeat perception technique with some social psychological approaches aimed at increasing self-attention of the subject (Duval & Wicklund, 1972; Wicklund, 1978). The subjects were 30 females, although it was thought that men would prove superior to women in cardiac perception (Katkin, 1985). Each session consisted of two identically structured parts, the only difference being that in one part the subjects performed the heartbeat discrimination task while facing a mirror (mirror condition), and in the other part, the mirror was turned away (no-mirror condition). The order of the two conditions was counterbalanced across subjects. The Whitehead-type (Whitehead *et al.*, 1977) heartbeat discrimination method was used, which showed significant improvement while facing a mirror than when the latter was absent (Fig. 13). Interestingly, presence of the mirror had no effect on the so-called heartbeat "tracking" performance used as a control (McFarland, 1975).

We consider this study (Weisz *et al.*, 1988) to be one of the far-reaching attempts among our experiments on viscerosomatic perception, since it might yield several explanations, some of them eventually leading to new vistas in the topic of this book. The most obvious explanation of the results relates to the function of attention. The mirror condition of each session enhanced self-attention,

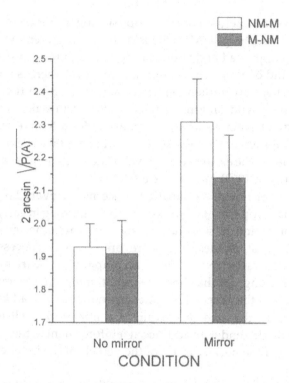

Figure 13. Correct heartbeat detections and standard errors of a group of subjects when looking (mirror) versys not looking (no mirror) in a mirror. NM-M, starting with no mirror; M-NM, starting with mirror condition. Reprinted from Weisz *et al.* (1988) with the permission of Cambridge University Press.

which might be a powerful tool for improving cardiac awareness. I must remind the reader that in the very first period of our human visceroceptive conditioning investigation, we already hypothesized, among other possibilities, that verbal or acoustic reinforcement of the duodenal or uterine stimuli might act through "whipping up" brain structures responsible for focused attention. Recent observations on unilateral sensory neglect suggest clinical means that are likely suitable for approaching the problem (Weisz, Soroker, Oksenberg, & Myslobodsky, 1995). At present, we lack a generally approved and valid conception as to the physiological background of attention. On the "macro" level, there is no doubt that both the Kluver–Bucy syndrome and the just-mentioned sensory neglect syndrome must have a close connection with the pathology of brain structures responsible for attentive behavior (e.g., some areas of the infratemporal and parietal cortex). On the "micro" level, the existence of "novelty" neurons or other detector cells (Sokolov, 1963) cannot be excluded either.

Another line of explanation concerns the everyday observation that people in general experience, beginning in early childhood, some kind of somatic and auditory rhythmic sensations, although most of these cases are preconscious processing of information (see Dixon, 1981), accompanying heart systoles. Thus, a lifelong peculiar operant conditioning process might be the basis and the cause of the phenomenon that we call *heartbeat perception*. In the case of looking in a mirror, the self-focused viewing might render an additional reinforcement to the constant pulsation of the neck arteries, of the vessels of the inner ear, and so on.

A third, alternative explanation of the mirror effect on heartbeat discrimination might be that, when facing a mirror, subjects undergo a higher level of emotional experience and that such an emotional arousal improved cardiac discrimination. It has been repeatedly demonstrated that higher emotional arousal leads to better heartbeat discrimination (Schandry & Specht, 1981; Katkin, 1985). The issue of the relation between emotion and visceral sensations fits in the framework of this chapter not only because of the mirror experiment, but also for more general and fundamental reasons. From the very beginning of our studies we became in some respects adherents of the Jamesian theory of emotion (see below) and emotional processes seem to be linked to the subdominant hemisphere.

Visceroception and Emotion

We are witnessing a peculiar renaissance of the theories concerning the genesis of emotions formulated separately by James (1907) in the United States and by Lange (1905) in Denmark. In the initial years of this rebirth, some of our own data pointed to the eventual importance of visceral input in the onset of emotions. In my earlier monograph (Ádám, 1967), it was formulated as follows: "Relying on our experimental data we presume that interoceptive impulses constitute an important afferent channel to cortical, limbic and mesencephalic structures governing emotional responses. These visceral signals seem to influence behaviour considerably both in man and animals, even though they become conscious in man only occasionally" (Appendix I, p. 181). In the years in which this statement was being formulated, we were already aware of the manifold means by which viscerosensory input could initiate or modify emotional reactions and even of the possibility that ongoing emotional behavior could alter the efficiency of visceroceptive signals. In the last quarter of a century, the above presumptions have been supported by many facts.

Originally it was Dell (1952) who advanced the principle that visceral afferents might exert an inhibiting influence on some brain activities associated with higher functions. Successive series of data emphasized the role of viscerosensory input in both directions. Some data from our laboratory documented that visceral stimulation induces synchronization of the EEG (Kukorelli & Juhász, 1976) and even "taming" of cats subject to the influence of ongoing hypothalamic rage (Kukorelli & Détári 1994). The calming, alleviating emotional effect of visceral afferent input was described and summarized in detail by Dworkin (1993). Notably, in his initial experiments on rats made hypertensive, he observed that high blood pressure exerts a wanted, reinforcing effect on the animals' behavior; in other words, the animals strive to remain hypertensive, as emotionally the situation seems to be "pleasant" for them. Dworkin, Filewich, Miller, Craigmyle, and Pickering (1979) interpreted their findings in such a way, namely, that arterial baroreceptor activity was a reinforcement of instrumental learning to reach a set point in the autonomic regulation of the hypertensive organism. In his important theoretical book just mentioned, (Dworkin, 1993) summarized his views about visceroreceptor mechanisms, regarding visceroception as a necessary tool in long-term physiological regulation, but not taking into due consideration the affective aspect of the baroreceptor mechanism that he had discovered. Contrary to the positive, "pleasant" emotional influence of visceral input discussed above, several findings, among others from our laboratory, seemed to point to an opposite mechanism elicited by GI visceroceptors in rats. Some findings documented that nonpainful visceral signals above a given threshold elicit aversive behavior, even discomfort (Bárdos, 1989). A peculiar kind of calibration was recommended; it was found that the mildly unpleasant "isovolemic" gut distention could be clearly distinguished from the "volumetric," marked elevation of the volume of the gut, which resulted in discomfort, occasionally in pain. The author relied on earlier data of others (Snowdon, 1970; Cabanac, 1971) in interpreting his findings. The apparently contrasting views and data on the dual influence of visceral signals, namely, in "switching on and off" emotions, more precisely in provoking "pleasant" or "unpleasant" affections, should be regarded as a matter of intensity of the visceral stimulus. In other words everything depends on the thresholds. Part IV of this monograph treats this problem.

Everyday observations as well as case histories in clinical psychology and medicine document that actual, ongoing emotional attitudes can be promptly modified, stopped, or increased by messages originating from visceroreceptors (e.g., Stern, Ray, & Davis, 1980). Emergency situations, such as the urgent need to void started by bladder or rectal mechanoreceptors, are obvious, albeit banal examples of such visceral alarm signals. Recall that one possible explanation of the findings of the mirror rexperiment—that when looking in a mirror, subjects improve their cardiac perception—is the higher level of emotional experience related to the "pleasure" of watching oneself in a mirror. All in all, the Jamesian conjecture can be revisited: Visceroception and emotion seem to be interwoven phenomena. Each might mutually influence the other in stimulating and inhibiting ways; each might be the motive and the effect of the other.

PART *IV*

Visceroception: Constituent of Special Senses

CHAPTER *10*

Visceroception
A Borderline Sensory System

If the reader were to consider that the preceding chapters had dealt exclusively with sensory phenomena other than visceroceptive ones—e.g., vision, audition, and, primarily, somatic sensory events—it would nonetheless be found that most if not all of the presumptions, results, and interpretations could be substituted by phenomena of the above-mentioned "classical" special senses. It has been clear from the very beginning of research in classical physiology and psychology of the special senses—i.e., from the initial achievements of such giants of sensory physiology as Helmholtz, Müller, and many others—that the fundamental laws of the special senses are common, in other words, that there has been and still is a reason for the existence of a general physiology of the special senses in research as well as in the curriculum of students in medicine, biology, and psychology. Most of the facts and concepts outlined above in the framework of visceral sensation and perception can and should be included in general physiology and even psychology.

Let me digress in introducing Part IV of this monograph. When I began teaching physiology for medical students in 1949, in

119

addition to the two or three textbooks in Hungarian then available, it was mainly the 10th edition of the Starling book (by Lovatt Evans) that served as our guiding text. The chapter on special senses was written by H. Hartridge. But neither his chapter, nor the many different reference (or textbook) chapters of the subsequent years up to the present, with very few exceptions, considered the physiology and psychology of visceral senses among the other well-known modalities. The reason can be guessed as far as vision, audition, olfaction, and gustation are concerned. These are all modalities with highly specialized, sophisticated sense organs, complexly developed over the long history of animal evolution. Such sense organs displayed an evolution in relation to their adequate single stimulus, such as electromagnetic waves, acoustic waves, or evaporized chemical substances, and consequently became "monomodal" organs. There is no need and no space here to make a complete list and enumerate all of the well-known highly organized "monomodal" receptor systems. I must emphasize instead that workers in the field of visceral sensation and perception, our group included, always draw the attention of those interested in of this topic that the closest homologues, or at least sense organs with features similar to visceroceptors, are the cutaneous end organs and proprioceptors as well as their central representations, in collective terms: the somatic receptors, pathways, and central projections. The somatosensory system is subordinated to the same laws and properties as the viscerosensory one, is a "multimodal" system of mechano-, thermo-, and pain receptors, like the visceroceptive apparatus, and last, but not least, the two systems are closely interwoven (see pp. 100, 104) and tightly overlap each other. We consider the exclusion of the viscerosensory function from the "ensemble" of the special senses to reflect an unjustified and irrational discriminatory attitude of some workers in the fields of classical physiology and experimental psychology. Guided probably by historical prejudice or an overemphasized anatomical standpoint, they continue to regard the viscerosensory system as an integral part of the autonomic nervous apparatus. If only homeostatic regulation is taken into consideration, such as regulation of cardiac activity, of the lungs, or of blood pressure, this view of the viscerosensory system as a constituent of the autonomic network can be justified. But, as firmly proved by a considerable number of good-quality review papers and monographs, some of them cited in this book, the visceral afferent apparatus acts along specific features, that go far beyond the boundaries of simply sensing some autoregulatory changes in homeostasis; it forms a homogeneous, although "multimodal," consistent sensory system. The peculiar features of the system are unequivocal, and distinguish it from other special senses:

1. The information collected by the system originates, as mentioned in Part II (pp. 58–59), from the main visceral structures, i.e., the cardiovascular, gastrointestinal, respiratory, and urogenital systems. In Part II (pp. 32–33) I tried also to fix the boundaries of the viscerosensory system in order to clarify the limitation toward humoral impact and toward nociceptive phenomena. I will not consider these restrictions here.

2. Other important features separating visceral sensitivity phenomena from other special sense systems are the so-called threshold problems, which hide the peculiar double-faced nature of viscerosensitive influence. These threshold relationships will be the topic of the next chapter.

3. Finally, a characteristic trait, equally significant, is related to cognition. We are not far from the actual situation if we consider visceral afferent signals as parts of a peculiar precognitive system, which under special conditions are able to switch into cognitive phenomena. Chapter 11 focuses on these precognitive aspects of visceral signals and on the premises of switching to cognitive ones.

Probably we are not far from reality if we attribute to the poorly differentiated, more-or-less simple and primitive histological structure (outlined in Part I, pp. 37–38) of the visceroreceptor system the fact that its signaling and information-transmitting activity remains in most cases a vague phenomenon, hard to identify. As repeatedly emphasized in the preceding chapters, especially under physiological conditions of everyday life, it is difficult to closely follow its consequences, which, except in some emergency situations, remain hidden events. From the very beginning of our psychophysiological research efforts on visceroception, we faced this peculiar latent nature of the internal stimuli. This meant that under "invasive" stimulation circumstances, we had to increase substantially the intensity of the stimuli applied, in order to achieve a given suprathreshold level needed for a well-defined response. In other words, we constantly witnessed the peculiar borderline character of the viscerosensory impact: depending on the intensity of this impact, it produced one kind of result or instead another kind, completely opposite the former. That is to say, depending on the thresholds, the "double-edged" nature of the system became obvious. In the next pages I examine one by one the different aspects of this "two-faced" system.

Homeostatic versus Behavioral (Extrahomeostatic) System

The main force behind this monograph, the *raison d'être* of our scientific thought, can be framed as our consistent pursuit of such domains of visceral afferent phenomena that proved to be beyond the well-studied and thoroughly described organ regulations, i.e., outside of homeostatic control in the strict meaning of the term. We called this sphere of events *behavioral* or *extrahomeostatic*, although in some cases they are certainly not behavioral, but homeostatic in the broad sense of the word. There is no room and no reason here to enumerate the homeostatic functions of visceroceptors as delicate sensors, triggers, and watchers of the stability of the *milieu interne* of the organism. Complete lists and thorough descriptions are readily available, there being no shortage of this kind of classical literature.

The other side of this double-faced system, the behavioral or extrahomeostatic aspect, is an issue of major concern to us for two reasons: (1) Certainly all consequences of visceral input that prove to be more than strictly organ-regulatory, and which constitute the main topic of the present work—e.g., perception through learning, emotional reactions—are likewise homeostatic in the broader sense of the term, since all such acquired behavioral events are serving the equilibrium of the organism as a whole. We called them *extrahomeostatic* or *behavioral* for practical, or rather didactic reason, to separate them from the strict regulatory side of the organs in Cannon's (1929) sense. (2) But we do not know at present the boundaries of one or the other part of the system; that is, under which circumstances does a viscerosensory train of signals constitute a message not only for a given organ to be regulated in a closed nervous loop, but also to higher central neuronal networks beyond this loop? Some of our data on the behavioral effects of carotid stimulation in dogs (Ádám, 1967) and other data suggest the presumption that the organ-regulatory and the behavioral aspects of visceral impact are not alternatives, but rather that the two effects are simultaneous. The distention of the carotid sinus by a balloon triggered blood pressure changes and conditional reflexes in synchrony. However, the supposition that the two effects are elicited by visceral impulses of different intensities along an intensity continuum cannot be excluded either. In the latter case the threshold intensity has to be quantified, but such a specification is not at all an easy task.

Arousing versus Sleep-Evoking System

In contrast to the difficulties encountered in the quantification of the borderline between organ-regulatory and behavioral
consequences of visceral impact, the determination of the threshold between the arousal-evoking and sleep-inducing effect of
visceral stimulation proved to be relatively successful. Kukorelli
and Juhász (1976) in our laboratory demonstrated that the weak-
intensity stimulation of the small intestine or of the splanchnic
nerve, in the previously operated chronic cat, evoked slow-wave
sleep both behaviorally and as seen on the EEG records. The
increase of the intensity of visceral stimulation to a given threshold
(the so-called viscero-somatomotor threshold) evoked behavioral
waking and desynchronized EEG.

This finding was later extended in a study of the effect of
vagal and splanchnic stimulation on hypothalamically induced
attack reactions of the cat (see Chapter 11) and compared with
the available literature. It was found that the data of Kukorelli
and Détári (1994) were in complete agreement with the above
electrophysiological results. In other studies, the same "double-
edged" character of visceral stimuli could be observed depending on the actual period of the sleep–wakefulness cycle (Kukorelli
& Juhász, 1983). In all of these experiments of Kukorelli's group
on cats with chronically implanted electrodes and isolated intestinal loops, the thresholds of "weak" and "strong" visceral stimuli were easily quantified. "Weak" stimulation meant that the
intensity of the square-wave impulses of 0.05 to 0.1-ms duration
reached only the threshold of the splanchnic afferents of large
diameter, the $A\beta$-fibers, whereas "strong" stimulation meant that
the same kind of electrical square-wave impulses reached the
thin splanchnic afferents too (Kukorelli & Juhász, 1983) (Fig. 14).
Consequently, these electrophysiological experiments, different
from observations on the homeostatic versus extrahomeostatic

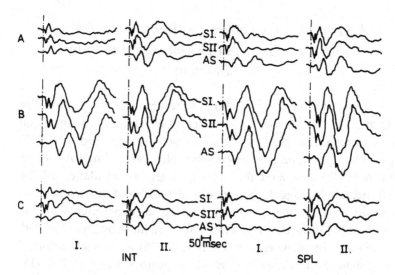

Figure 14. Averaged evoked potentials of the cat from the somatosensory (SI, SII) and associative (AS) cortical areas to weak (I) and strong (II) electrical stimulation of the intestines (INT) and of the splanchnic nerve (SPL) during wakefulness (A), slow-wave (B) and paradoxical (C) sleep. Reprinted from Kukorelli and Juhász (1976) with the kind permission of Elsevier Science - NL.

influence of visceral afferents described in the previous chapter, render a more-or-less exact threshold measurement possible. And as a result of such a quantification, the alternative character of the visceral input becomes clear: In contrast to homeostatic–behavioral pairs, where, as outlined above, both effects can be hypothesized as acting simultaneously, here, in the case of desynchronizing–synchronizing pairs, such a simultaneity is not possible. The visceral signals will act in one way or the other, evoking either arousal or sleep, and simultaneous impact will not be possible, given that the rest of the physiological parameters remain unchanged.

A System Evoking Negative Motivation and Stress Induction versus Positive Motivation and Stress Reduction

The "double-faced" nature of the viscerosensory impact in its motivational aspect was mentioned in reference to emotional phenomena and their interrelations with visceral input (p. 113) and when discussing our electrophysiological findings. Although Koch (1932) described the taming effect of stimulation of the carotid area in dogs shortly after the discovery of the reflexogenic carotid area by Hering (1923), the crucial experiments on the motivational effect of visceral stimuli were those by Dworkin *et al.* (1979) and by Kukorelli and Juhász (1976) in our laboratory. I described the findings of Dworkin's group above (pp. 113–114) emphasizing that Dworkin included later (1993) their data into the framework of a general theory on the role of learned reactions in physiological regulations. The key investigation of Kukorelli and co-workers examined the effect of splanchnic and vagal (i.e., visceral afferent) weak-intensity stimulation on (1) aggressive behavior evoked by direct electrical irritation of the hypothalamic "rage centers" and on (2) the sleep–wakefulness cycle modified by hypothalamic stimulation. As already mentioned, it was found that weak visceral input significantly increases the latency of aggressive reaction and increases the time-share of slow-wave sleep and paradoxical sleep in the sleep–wakefulness cycle. Thus, the calming, taming influence of these weak visceral stimuli can be hypothesized (Fig. 15). Regarding the inverse effects, namely, the influences of more intensive visceral impulses on motivated behavior, a whole series of findings, such as those cited in the discussion on aversive emotions (p. 114), seem to establish such an irritating, annoying, stress-inducing result (e.g., Snowdon, 1970; Garcia, Hankins, & Rusiniak, 1974). We believe that the unpleasant effects of intensive visceral signals are more-or-less

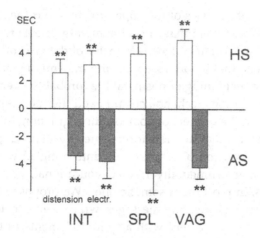

Figure 15. Effects of intestinal (INT), splanchnic (SPL), and vagal (VAG) electrical stimulation on the biting latency of predatory behavior due to hypothalamic stimulation in the cat. The visceral mechanical (distention) or electrical (electr.) stimuli were either hypnogenic (HS) or arousing (AS). HS was delivered for 5 min and AS 10 sec prior to hypothalamic stimulation. Reprinted from Kukorelli and Détári (1994) with the kind permission of Elsevier Science - NL.

evident even in everyday psychological self-observation, in clinical practice, and elsewhere. It suffices to consider the discomfort after overeating, or the uneasiness following distention of the bladder or rectum. The taming and irritating influences of viscerosensory stimuli exclude the other; so that one state of motivation locks out the other, as we have seen in the case of desynchronizing versus synchronizing twin effects.

A System Sending Inherent versus Learned Messages

In the course of aligning the different aspects of the "double-edged," Janus-faced viscerosensory system, I must revisit the issues and controversies of the apparatus that was the subject of Chapter 8. It was there that I listed many arguments reinforcing the dual, inborn versus learned character of the visceral input. It will be recalled that inborn reception and transmission must exist from the very beginning of postnatal life (probably in embryonic life too), since these mechano-, chemo-, and thermoreceptive signals constitute the triggers of homeostatic regulation. In all probability, after birth they are transformed step by step, but probably very rapidly, into complex sensations, intermingled with classically or/and instrumentally formed conditional, i.e., learned, components, in most cases somatic ones. We proposed the term *inherent* for such elementary messages, which were already "contaminated" to some extent with acquired elements in the early period of ontogenesis.

From this brief description, it is quite evident that, contrary to both the arousing versus sleep-evoking and the stress-inducing versus stress-reducing dual aspects of visceroception in which one state of the twin condition excludes the other state, the inherent versus learned characters of this two-faced apparatus do not exclude each other. In our opinion, as for the homeostatic versus behavioral double-featured aspects outlined above (p. 122), the two sides postulate each other. Namely, inborn sensory visceromechanisms become transformed into more intricate inherent activities, which will be converted into complex learned sensations and even perceptions (see p. 89).

A System Sending Nonconscious versus Conscious Messages

The last aspect in this brief enumeration of the double-faced, borderline character of the viscerosensory system concerns nonconscious versus conscious phenomena. In the early period of my scientific education, being a follower of the Pavlovian and later of the Thorndikeian–Skinnerian trends, I tried to avoid the use of terms such as *consciousness*, and instead employed the terms *verbally reportable* and *nonreportable*. Later, after completing the series of experiments wherein we applied duodenal distention and uterine stimulation as visceral signals and reinforced these "nonreportable" visceral messages by simultaneous verbal information about the onset of the internal stimuli (see pp. 96–97), I realized suddenly that the twin terms *nonconscious* and *conscious* are both theoretically and practically indispensable. Since the advent of thorough experimental investigation of sensory mechanisms, all researchers have acknowledged that a number of sensory messages reached the brain without being consciously perceived (Fig. 16). Nevertheless, scientists are not unanimous

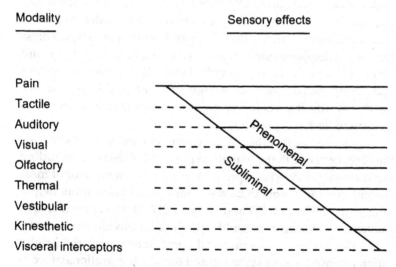

Figure 16. Dixon's ranking of conscious ("phenomenal") and nonconscious ("subliminal") aspects of different sensory modalities. He put "visceral interoceptors" at the bottom, displaying the largest "subliminal" sensory effect. From Dixon (1981). Published with the kind permission of Wiley and Sons, Limited.

regarding a general and validated theory of the unconscious and the conscious. In Chapter 2, I touched on the problem, and emphasized that wakefulness and awareness are prerequisites of consciousness, but not identical with it. The absence of wakefulness precludes any conscious perception. But not all sensory processes reach consciousness even in the wakeful state.

One of the most debated issues seems to be the relation of conscious phenomena with their verbal expression. According to a popular theory, consciousness is the simultaneous presence in higher brain structures of signals originating from primary environmental stimuli and those due to abstract verbalized signals. Thus, consciousness can be defined as the sum of multiple sensations and other mental phenomena (e.g., retrieved memory contents, emotional reactions) in a given moment. In this sense, the conscious state is the result of the synchronous activity of several cortico-subcortical units integrated into a single functional system. In this aspect, verbal expression can be regarded as part of such a unified system. On the other hand, mute persons speechless from birth display evident signs of conscious sensory, motor, and other phenomena and some evident visceral conscious sensations and perceptions do not have any semantic or semiotic equivalents; in other words, it is likely that not every conscious experience has a clear-cut verbal expression.

A survey of theories on the nature of consciousness reveals the absence of one that adequaty explains all of the facts, including our own data on visceroception. A common denominator of most current theories seems to be the principle of dissociation. Beginning with Spinoza (1677) and Leibnitz (1765) up to Freud (1964), thinkers and researchers could not imagine individual consciousness other than as a hierarchical construction with the bright, rational consciousness at the top and the obscure irrational unconsciousness at the bottom. Today, we refer to several compartments of conscious and nonconscious contents coordinated beside, not above or below, each other. In a given period of time, usually some of these compartments dominate as others remain in the background; in another time period, different compartments are transformed into "bright" and the rest into "dim" ones; and so on. It was Pierre Janet who described the compartments of consciousness with scientific rigor. He wrote about "dissociation" of mind (in contrast to "association") and examined in detail some double or even triple personalities revealed in hypnosis. He proposed the term *subconscious* instead of *unconscious* introduced by von Hartmann. Janet's conception deeply influenced Freud's theories about "preconscious," "unconscious" and "conscious." There is no opportunity here to appreciate or criticize these early principles. More recently, Hilgard (1965) renewed the old theories and proposed calling them *neodissociation* principles. In his view, the different compartments of consciousness are present in every healthy personality, but due to some well-functioning control systems they cooperate with each other. One of these control mechanisms, the so-called "hidden observer" (corresponding to the "ego" or "self" of other theories), integrates the divided compartments and facilitates the crosswalk among different closed psychical "boxes."

Accepting the compartment principle of consciousness, there is at present no evidence establishing the location of any function of the mind in one of these dissociated "boxes." Consequently, we are unable to assign nonconscious or conscious visceral sensations to well-defined compartments. We can only guess that the nonreportable viscerosensory input of one dim compartment is able to switch to "bright" one (i.e., conscious one) via special mechanisms. Earlier I outlined two such processes that in all probability facilitate or even trigger separately or jointly the crosswalk through "passageways" from one compartment (e.g., nonconscious sensations) to another (e.g., conscious sensations or perceptions), namely, the mechanism of attention and that of conditioning, learning (see pp. 128–129). These two mechanisms are capable of highlighting those dim mental phenomena that

Table 3. The "Janus-Faced" Double Influence on Five Different Aspects of Behavior of Visceroceptive Impact Represented along an Intensity Continuum from Zero to Nociceptive Intensity

NOCICEPTIVE INTENSITY

COVERT OR OVERT INFLUENCE ON BEHAVIORAL (PSYCHOLOGICAL) PHENOMENA	EVOKING AROUSAL = DESYNCHRONIZING EEG	EVOKING NEGATIVE MOTIVATION, ENLARGING REACTIVITY TO STRESS, AGRESSIVENESS	NATURAL INHERENT SIGNAL DETECTION, DISCRIMINATION	SENDING CONSCIOUS, REPORTABLE MESSAGES IF LEARNED OR SOMATICALLY REINFORCED
ONLY AFFERENT LOOP OF ORGAN REGULATIONS IN HOMEOSTASIS	EVOKING SLOW WAVE SLEEP = SYNCHRONIZING EEG	EVOKING POSITIVE MOTIVATION, REDUCING REACTIVITY TO STRESS, TAMING	SIGNAL DETECTION, DISCRIMINATION BY LEARNING	SENDING NON-CONSCIOUS, NON-REPORTABLE MESSAGES. PERCEPTION BY SOMATIC MEDIATION OR BY LEARNING

ZERO INTENSITY

seem to be important at the given time from the point of view of cognition and to eliminate those that seem unimportant or redundant. Attention and learning are consequently the main tools in the service of rendering conscious (i.e., verbally reportable) previously nonconscious (i.e., nonreportable) events. In this respect I again refer to the Preface and the attempt made there to define "perception" and to distance it from "sensation." Quoting Freeman (1981, 1983) and later Mountcastle (1980), it becomes clear that we consider conscious experience as an essential component of perception, but negligible in the case of sensation, which might be virtually nonconscious as well as conscious (see pp. 8, 13–15).

Summing up this chapter on different borderline aspects of visceral messages, viscerosensory signals act along an intensity continuum in the middle of which a given "threshold" must be approximated, determined, even quantified, since precisely this "threshold" is the limit between one kind of response to a weak visceral stimulus and another kind of response to a stronger visceral impact. Unfortunately, even the rough approximation of such a border line seems to raise difficulties (except the threshold between desynchronizing and synchronizing EEG and motivational reactions), as outlined one by one in this brief survey (Table 3).

The Janus-faced nature of visceroception is remarkable since it displays at the same time: (1) a common denominator with the other, classical sense organs such as the visual, auditory, and tactile systems, which also act along given intensity continua and thresholds, and (2) a line of demarcation, a specific distinction opposed to classical special senses, which do not collect the majority of their information from the low-intensity, covert *milieu interne* as does the viscerosensory system.

CHAPTER *11*

Visceroception and Cognition

The main task of the present work cannot be accomplished without confronting viscerosensory phenomena with those higher processes of the brain that are nowadays included in the collective term *cognitive events*. The term *Erkenntnistheorie* was introduced by Reinhold (1789) and became popular, even fashionable, in the last 15–20 years due to the rapid development of information theory, of psycholinguistics, and of research in artificial intelligence. The word *cognition* (knowledge) has two main meanings: (1) representation in the brain of an object or a process from the environment, concrete or abstract, by perception, concept formation, or imagination, and (2) understanding of that object or process and placing it in the framework of the system of objects or processes already known. This rather alienated, abstract paraphrase of the "overwinded" term covers, in our opinion, very realistic phenomena that should be formulated in the following questions: (1) Does information arriving in the brain from internal organs through (conscious) perceptive phenomena form cognitive schemes, or maps? (2) is the mind capable of identifying and naming the internal information so as to arrange them in their proper place in the mental image network? I will try to approach these questions

135

Close-up: The Placebo Problem

Modeling the role of visceral signals in triggering cognitive processes can be done by considering the *placebo* phenomenon. It is well known that the current fulminant development of medical treatment and pharmacological knowledge has been accompanied by very powerful *expectations* of the general community. It is no wonder that *new* drugs or surgical interventions exert, besides their proper curing effect, an *additional* beneficial healing in most patients. The latter influence is due to the *demands* of the subjects. The sarcastic remark, attributed to the great French physiologist Trousseau, that we should cure rapidly as many patients as possible with a new drug as long as it still preserves its healing power, hides an elementary truth, namely, the cognitive disposition of people in the direction of their recovery and their trustful anticipation of the new treatment. Pharmaceutical companies and pharmacologists are very aware that a newly introduced and advertised drug always shows extra success in the first months or even years of its introduction . This superior achievement is due in all probability to the expectations of the public, i.e., to an anticipatory mental phenomenon. The latter phenomenon is probably the only effect common to all medicaments.

I regard the existence of such an anticipatory behavior as the very essence of the placebo effect. This same anticipatory attitude may be the background for the positive healing effect of numerous pseudoremedies, sham treatments, false devices, and the like unfortunately so popular in Central Europe and elsewhere. The latter treatments in all probability trigger *mental anticipation* awaiting action in the higher faculties of the brain.

Several trends in personality psychology are in agreement with the assumption that a peculiar *mental image of the self* is always in the course of formation and perfection, beginning in early infancy and continuing throughout life. This mental scheme or image of our own personality, in the cognitive psychological sense of the word, is constructed by learning, or rather "overlearning," in most cases as the representation of a *healthy, intact* self, since we imagine ourselves from early childhood as unhurt, sound persons. I have no doubt whatsoever that the preservation, maintenance, and eventual restoration of the integrity and unharmed nature of this image is one of the main goals (if not *the* main goal) of individual existence. Consequently, any tool, real or sham, seems suitable to satisfy our expectations for the restoration of a brain map that reflects the intactness of our physical and mental condition in case of a real or threatening illness. The cognitive representation of the self is in all probability a *dominant* scheme, forcing its way to the surface whenever the imagined integrity of the private personality is endangered. Terms such as *self-esteem, self-assertion, self-deceit, self-love, self-pity,* and many others very likely reflect such a prevailing mental image.

Any stimulus can serve as trigger and initiator reestablishing the equilibrium of a disturbed cognitive self-picture. The term *placebo-factor* refers to a given external intervention into the regulatory function of an organism that not only is efficient, i.e., acts at the proper site of the disturbed organ or system, but that also acts on the cognitive faculties of the brain, i.e., in addition to influencing the organism it also *pleases* (the Latin word *placebo* is the future tense of the verb *placēre*, which means "to please"); in other words, it should exert not only an organic, but also a *mental* influence on the medicative activity. According to general belief, the term originated from the Latin version of the Bible (Vulgate), namely, Psalm 116:9 states: "Placebo Domino in regione vivorum" ("I will please the Lord in the World of the living"). I must emphasize that, contrary to the general view underestimating the placebo effect (a usual medical statement being, "this is merely a placebo phenomenon"), this impact is a powerful reality, mobilizing the reserve powers of the recovering organism under the guidance of the dominant cognitive self-representation of the brain. In other words, the placebo influence not only pleases, but also proves to be efficacious too. The placebo effect is thus a real phenomenon acting on the brain, but one that physicians, psychologists, and most researchers in the behavioral sciences are not aware of.

Such disregard of the placebo phenomenon is not of secondary importance, since the effect, I predict, will achieve much significance in the near future not only in various therapeutic directions, but also in our proper topics of interest, such as psychosomatic medicine, visceral learning, and visceral perception.

Regarding the *mechanisms* of action of the placebo effect, we are unfortunately far from possessing documented and validated data. Many researchers believe, as do we, that the two main classes of associative learning, i.e., (1) *classical* and (2) *operant conditioning* paradigms, may be the main tools in the formation of the mental cognitive maps described above. It is well known that the temporal contiguity of two or more stimuli evoking genetically given responses, i.e., the synchronous course of two or more inborn reflexes, will result in the formation of a new reaction, in which the biologically dominant side will constitute the reinforcement, whereas the less dominant one either will form the signal (in the case of classical conditioning), or will be transformed into an acquired response (in the case of instrumental, or operant, conditioning).

As background in the case of classical conditioning, the warning stimulus or reminding signal (CS) appears simultaneously with a biologically important stimulus (US), evoking a well-recognizable physiological change in the activity of some organ or system and at the same time forming a mental image of that modification of the system. After several repetitions of this simultaneous appearance of the CS with the US, the application of the CS without the reinforcing US will be able to evoke a similar, or even identical, physiological change as originally elicited by the US. And, what is even more important from the cognitive standpoint, the CS will be able to activate the mental scheme formed during the previous pairings of the CS with the US. The coupling of the Pavlovian principles of conditioning with the principles of formation of mental representations, outlined briefly above, was initiated originally by Peter Anokhin (1968), associate of Pavlov. He regarded the already elaborated conditional responses as "preliminary reflections of reality" in the higher brain centers, i.e., as real mental images. It is easy to recognize in the just-drafted mechanism the emergence of the placebo phenomenon following a reminding stimulus or cue (CS), which happened to be reinforced previously, sometimes on a single occasion, sometimes repeatedly, with a powerful impact causing physiological changes in the organism (US). The pairing trials resulted in the elaboration of the typical placebo effect provoked this time by the cue stimulus (CS) alone.

Turning now to operant, or instrumental, conditioning, this paradigm is similarly suitable for explaining the emergence of a placebo phenomenon reflecting the formation of a cognitive brain scheme. In this variant of associative learning, the mental representation of a strong reinforcing stimulus, in most cases a reward, in some cases a punishment, is paired with an accidentally produced physiological change. The simultaneous repeated appearance of the reinforcement with the organ change originally produced only by chance, will result in the acquirement and storage, i.e., in the learning process, of the same functional organ modification. The latter, consequently, will switch from being an accidental phenomenon into a regularly appearing learned event, which, in cognitive terms, means that its mental representation has been elaborated due to the reinforcing associations. This type of associative learning, originally described by Edward Lee Thorndike (1898) as "the law of effect"and later developed by B. F. Skinner (1938), can be regarded as the background mechanism of the placebo effect as well.

According to the principles of cognitive psychology, the mental representation of the above-described acquired activity is in all probability an integrated, holistic phenomenon. In other words, the placebo effect can be regarded as a "Gestalt" in the original meaning of the term coined by Ehrenfels (1890). In this sense, the newly created mental scheme, formed by associative learning, will merge into the already existing powerful Gestalt of the healthy and intact self-scheme outlined above. Thus, the newly formed placebo image will serve as a peculiar *reinforcement* of the already existing and permanently functioning unimpaired self-pattern. More exactly, the placebo intervention will trigger the restoration of the self-picture of the unhurt and sound organism that all of us carefully preserve from our early childhood. A series of experimental and clinical arguments seem to prove the existence of this "intactness" image of the self. It will suffice to mention the so-called "phantom feelings," "phantom pain,"or "phantom movements." Weeks, months, or even years after the complete amputation of a limb, the individual experiences feelings originating from the missing limb, is able to localize the source of those feelings or pain, and can initiate "movements" starting from the amputated arm or leg. In these cases, the phantom phenomena are obviously taking place in the brain areas preserving the projection of the given limb and are sending messages from those mental representations.

The placebo effects, contrary to the impacts of the real curing interventions, are merely *temporary* phenomena. After days, weeks, or months of expectations, the *plus effect* of anticipation diminishes step by step and, finally, fades away, provided it is not reinforced by the real medication. The curing effects of the medicative interventions, of course, will persist. Thus, the placebo phenomenon follows the Pavlovian rules of *extinction* of a conditional reflex: If not reinforced from time to time, i.e., if the placebo stimulus (the CS) is repeatedly applied merely by itself, without the occasional application of the real treatment (the US), the learned response gradually diminishes and finally disappears.

The placebo phenomenon is a general human feature, and apparently there is no way to "escape" its influence under certain circumstances. However, we don't really know what those circumstances are. Cognitive and experimental medical sciences, although able to describe and even to specify some kinds of placebo effects, have not elucidated their mechanisms or their detailed backgrounds. I will briefly enumerate three of these unsolved problems.

1. We don't know anything about the "placebo personality" or "temperament." The cognitive process via associative learning, outlined above, is characteristic of every human being, but the randomly examined human groups display a peculiar statistical distribution. About 20 to 40% of those examined show a high degree of placebo sensitivity, and another 20 to 40% a mean susceptibility. Our earlier data showed that placebo sensitivity and responsiveness to hypnosis are different typological entities, but other personality relations are unknown.

2. We are ignorant about the type and number of physiological and pathophysiological functions that are subject to placebo responses and about those systems that eventually might be exempt from this mental influence. A considerable amount of data point to the high sensitivity of the cardiovascular and digestive systems to mental interventions, i.e., to close brain–internal organ relationships, e.g., to their learning abilities. Certain visceral functions, such as the activity of the sweat glands, are almost unprecedented examples of systems that are constantly under psychological control. But the entire catalogue of physiological processes easily influenced by mental interventions as well as their detailed mechanisms of action are far from known.

3. The efferent and—what is the focus of this book—the *afferent* pathways going to and coming from the internal organs, subject to placebo phenomena, together with their central neuronal representations and especially their *mode of activity* remain to be revealed. The first part of this book touched on some anatomical, histological, and physiological details concerning viscerosensory functions, but I am convinced that such data are too rough and not appropriate or relevant yet to tackle the complex psychophysiological phenomena that were discussed here.

without penetrating into the philosophical or even psychological depth of the cognition problem.

Protopathic and Epicritic Systems

Neurologists still appreciate and apply in their theoretical and clinical activities the proposals of Henry Head (1920), who at the turn of the twentieth century in then-famous self-experiments tried to classify the basic forms of human somatic sensations. He instructed his colleagues to perform a rather simple surgical intervention on his arm, namely, to cut the nervus cutaneus antebrachii lateralis on one forearm. With this surgery, the area of the skin innervated by this nerve became completely anesthetized, while the neighboring skin surface, innervated by the nervus cutaneus antebrachii medialis, became hypersensitive to thermal and to noxious stimuli. Starting from this self-experiment, Head had drafted his principle of classification still in use in somatosensory neurology in most European and even American hospitals. He proposed the term *protopathic sensibility* for the function of the more ancient, less differentiated system of carrying thermal and pain messages from the periphery through spinal and bulbar relay neurons to higher thalamic and cortical networks. This diffuse apparatus is unable to precisely detect and recognize nociceptive or thermal stimuli in space and time, its memory storage also being unarticulated and global. Its emotional influence is vivid and powerful: Acute affective reactions accompany both thermal and noxious messages, the latter always being unpleasant. [Pribram (1971) proposed calling the system *protocritic*].

In contrast to this system, *epicritic sensibility* was proposed for the phylogenetically more recent sensory pathways carrying precisely discriminable, well-articulated tactile, pressure, and movement messages. Originally, Head used the term only to mark delicate, well- localizable haptic sensations (hence the term *epi-*

critic), whereas later it was usually applied to name all other sensibilities (e.g., vision, audition) that transmit subtle, well-structured and definable information. This classification, already considered outdated 30–40 years ago, underwent a peculiar renaissance in the last decade, since it became clear in the present era of cognitive boom that the category of epicritic sensibility includes all of those messages from the external world that are able to create definite representations, so-called cognitive maps or schemes in the brain. From the purport of this work, it is obvious that epicritic sensibility does not match visceral perception at least in normal everyday life. As emphasized repeatedly in the preceding chapters, sophisticated conditioning or signal-detection paradigms had to be applied in order to compel our subjects to pay special attention to signals arriving from the abdomen or heart. Of course, the same conditioning or signal-detection techniques are often applied in studying auditory, visual, somatosensory, and other subthreshold, hidden phenomena, eventually even unreportable ones, but in the case of viscerosensory events, except for emergency or urgency, "natural" conscious (i.e., epicritic) visceral perceptions without learning or forced choice do not occur at all, visceral sensations remaining always in the shadow of dim, diffuse sensibility.

It follows from the foregoing that we include visceral perception in the category of protopathic sensory activities. As known from the relevant literature (e.g., Dixon, 1981; Weiskrantz, 1986), nonconscious or preconscious sensory processes may also form mental images, and some kind of dim, long-term memory storage may exist. But such brain schemata are less "grained," rough and diffuse, as demonstrated in the case of thermal and nociceptive messages. Obviously, viscerosensory nonconscious and even conscious phenomena belong to the protopathic class. It is our assumption that all characteristics of the viscerosensory apparatus discussed in the foregoing chapters point without exception to its protopathic nature. Its input to the telencephalon is poorly localizable and the messages are hardly discriminable, not to mention the very special features of its sensations amply related in this essay. Even anatomically, similarly to the main protopathic systems like the nociceptive and temperature-carrying pathways, visceral signals are carried for the most part (see pp. 58–62 for spinal afferent fibers and tracts) by extralemniscal bundles through the spinal cord and brainstem. Finally, from the point of view of evolution, similarly to the ancient protective function of nociception, visceroception is regarded as a phylogenetically and ontogenetically ancestral apparatus "losing" its priorities in its competition with exteroception (e.g., vision, audition) in the struggle for survival (see also pp. 25–27).

On the Doorsteps of Cognition

Cognitive psychologists do not deny the mental representations of protopathic messages, whether nonconscious or conscious. Both pain and heat (cold) signals usually initiate hardly definable, but sometime long-lasting memory traces. Such long-term memory contents are at the same time mostly unstructured, unrecognizably blurred, faded. Our own human data indicate that this is precisely the case with the visceral input, even if consciously perceived.

In the foregoing chapters we have seen that perception of changes occurring inside the body, near the mucous membrane or the muscular layer of the hollow viscera or the endothelia of the arteries, can probably be learned or improved by conditioning. In our opinion, we observed in those experiments the same perceptive phenomena that occur when the neonate learns to detect and to discriminate external visual, somatosensory, or auditory cues. Hebb (1949) proposed, and later rendered it very likely, that the human capacity for recognizing and identifying patterns in vision represents a very long process. He quoted Senden's (1932), who reported that humans with congenital cataract initially after surgery are unable to identify or to discriminate a circle, square, triangle, sphere, or cube. The initial discrimination between a cockscomb and a horse tail is a difficult task for these patients. Mishkin and Appenzeller's (1987) data on tachistoscopic recognition errors reinforce these findings. Consequently, the course of perceptual learning in man and other animals must be a gradual process as demonstrated also in animals reared in darkness (Hubel & Wiesel, 1963). Even the most intelligent human patients need months and even years to learn to precisely identify simple objects. Investigators seem to be unanimous on this point.

As repeatedly emphasized in this essay, in contrast to the perceptive processes exploring the external world, the messages originating from the internal milieu generally remain below the conscious level. Our internal sensitivity has very little, if any, chance in the normal course of life to detect, recognize, identify, discriminate and at last label visceral changes, because there is no need to do so, except for a few emergency situations outlined repeatedly. Broadbent (1958) and others have shown that the individual possesses at a given time a limited quantum of attention in the framework of his or her awareness, or wakefulness. In adults (but not infants, see p. 27), this attention is directed in far greater degree toward external cues, not internal ones. The situation may be reversed in extreme urgency conditions, such as starvation or high bladder or rectal tension. It seems to be quite different in the case of so-called "beliefs" or "naive theories" about various aspects of our bodies in symptom reports, as shown by Pennebaker (1982). Following several kinds of imaginational processes, each individual creates over the course of years certain ideas of how the organism works. These beliefs are deeply influenced by the cultural and social environments of the subjects and also by some illusions (see "Visceral Illusions," pp. 149–153), which in their totality can be considered as backgrounds of these symptom reports tested by Leventhal's and Pennebaker's groups and many others.

It may be assumed that normal internal perception stops ontogenetically in early childhood on the way to "growing up," but the possibility of perceiving, and identifying visceral signals is "built in" in the neuronal circuitry of every human (and animal) brain. Granit (1959) attached great importance to the sensory learning process as a possibility for individuals to better adapt to the needs of the environment. This Darwinian rule of adaptation through learning was described by Granit as the "law of relevance," giving as an example the color-detection and discrimination learning by the cat. This species is known as a poor detector of colors, but in a relevant, or wanted, situation, under the pressure of the environmental stimuli, can be taught to detect and discriminate colors. In our opinion, this Darwinian rule of adaptation is not far from the idea of "ecological interoception" proposed by Pennebaker (1995). In his paper, starting from the concepts of Gibson (1979) on the role of ecological factors in psychophysics, Pennebaker described his experiments on cardiac perception that attempted to "disentangle situational and physiological cues." It was found that self-reports on heart rate show an error of 51% due to situational beliefs, which nonetheless proved to be a more acceptable estimate than beliefs on finger temperature, which showed an error of 68.3% in comparison with the actual values (Fig. 17). Consequently, symptom reports seem to depend to a high degree on environmental, situational cues as emphasized by Granit.

Some cognitive scientists earlier put a sign of equality between epicritical memory and cognitive maps in the brain. The extreme "Gestaltists" and other followers of the cognitive representation conceptions had denied the possibility of formation of topographical patterns in the brain following internal sensations. More recently, however, due to research in the area of preconscious processing (Dixon, 1981), cognition without verbalization (Weiskrantz, 1986), and preattentive perception (Julesz, 1987), the assumption of production of protopathic schemata in the brain seems to be validated. Thus, conscious awareness, epicritical pre-

A

Heart Rate

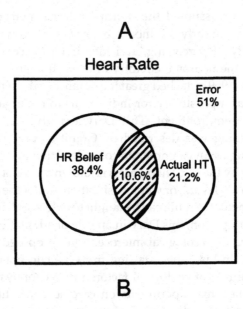

B

Finger Temperature

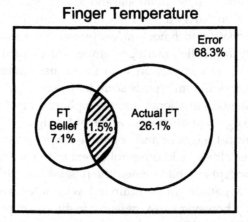

Figure 17. Pennebaker's diagram on the proportions between beliefs and actual values of heart rate and finger temperature self-reports. From Pennebaker (1995). Published with the kind permission of *Peter Lang, GmbH*. Frankfurt am Main.

cise and fine analysis of the environment, is no longer regarded as a precondition of the creation of some holistic representation, i.e., a sort of protopathic cognitive map in the brain. Our own research does not exclude such a possibility either. For instance, young right-handed subjects who happen to be good heartbeat detectors without any training in our laboratory, have improved their detection ability by activating their nondominant hemisphere. These findings can be interpreted to mean that people experience periodically throughout their lifetime some degree of heartbeat rhythmicity. Namely, we store rhythmic mechanical phenomena coming from the heart, combined with those periodic beats arriving from the auditory and somatosensory systems. Thus, we acquire a peculiar "time pattern," probably stored in the right hemisphere, which can be retrieved from that location when needed. Looking in a mirror—a powerful emotional stimulus of self-focused attention—enhances heartbeat detection. The above-mentioned data allude to the possibility of a holistically stored "visceral memory" in the brain by means of many years of "overlearning." The same phenomenon can be conjectured in the case of anal sensitivity. Under pressure of the social environment, people learn and store a definite pattern as to excrement in the rectum. Fine discriminative ability is stored and retrieved whenever needed about the physical state of the feces or the gases. Intensity and topographic discrimination ability of different intestinal stimuli has been repeatedly reported by our group over the last 25 years, both in animals and in humans. All of these findings encourage the view about a very rudimentary, although real "cognitive visceral map," stored in the course of very long periods of learning. The conjecture about the process of "overlearning" as a possible mechanism of long-term visceral memory has triggered another supposition: It seems to me highly possible that the analogues of visual, haptic, auditive, and other illusions thoroughly studied in the psychology of special senses are present also in the world of visceral perceptions. Most authors agree that illusions are the results of rigid, completely fixed and overlearned schemata in the brain (Révész, 1956). We know of no reason to exclude visceral perceptive phenomena from the rich array of sensory illusions. The "abnormal" perceptions of "normal" physiological changes in the esophagus (e.g., gastroesophageal reflux disease, globus sensation; see Bradley & Richter, 1996) may be the results of such "visceral illusions" which can serve even as bases of symptom reports (Pennebaker, 1982).

Visceral Perception and Cognitive Style

Chapter 9 underlined the importance of hemispheric lateralization in visceral (and viscerosomatic) information processing. Numerous findings on the preponderant role of the subdominant hemisphere in viscerosensory perception were presented, and described our experimental approach, namely, the application of tests to reveal the cognitive style of our experimental subjects, and presumed the role of some gender differences. Males who displayed a preference of leftward eye movements, i.e., who were subdominant (right) hemisphere preferents, were more accurate in solving spatial than verbal tasks. Also, it is generally validated that an individual's preference either for a spatial, or for a verbal cognitive problem-solving task is a quite firm and stable personality trait. This means that a person's cognitive style has a preference either toward verbal or toward spatial. Males are considered more spatial, and females, rather verbal. Another line of studies revealed that females report far more symptoms than do males and visit physicians to a greater extent (Pennebaker, 1982). In our study of the relations of visceral input and cognition, we decided to approach the reverse problem too, namely, whether visceral signals alter cognitive style. With spatial and verbal cognitive standards as our starting points, we made an attempt to answer this question.

Close-up: Visceral Illusions?

"Our past influences our present and our future": this statement is fully valid in the domain of human special senses. It is well known that we never perceive images, sounds, touched objects, flavors, or odors exactly in their "naked" physical or chemical reality. A certain degree of distortion is always present in all of our perceptions. These "mistakes" in perception are not in the least abnormal or anomalous phenomena: Their presence is as regular and steady as the process of perceiving itself. Probably Lipps (1897) was the first researcher to investigate the mental principles and the psychological backgrounds of these distortions. He used the term *Täuschungen* (= delusions, misses, or misinformation) to name these false events, but the notion of "illusions" gained ground in the psychological literature.

According to Lipps and some other researchers of the same era (Schumann, 1900; Benussi, 1914), the sensory illusions have to be regarded as regular and normal phenomena of the perceptive process that are always operating distorting the objectively existing reality in a subjectively misshapen way. Révész (1934) analyzed in detail the common laws of the illusions of different modalities and demonstrated three psychological tendencies in the course of formation of illusions, namely: *shaping, altering,* and *rectifying* trends.

1. The *shaping* tendency constitutes the implementation of the cognitive mental image (see p. 159) in the process of perception. Since the long-term memory of the brain stores a given amount of schemes of different sensory modalities accumulated in the permanent storage, it is only too obvious that these retained brain patterns will assist in perceiving. A collection of examples is fairly rich concerning almost every classical modality of the senses. The root of every one of these involves constructing (i.e., "shaping") an integrated picture, pattern, or scheme from fragments of reality perceived, in other words to prepare a *coherent* mental representation from little pieces of sensations. In all probability, the brain is applying in these cases its tendency to form gestalts (Ehrenfels, 1890).

2. The *altering* tendency constitutes the most intriguing feature of the illusions since it comprises the *distorting* side of the whole misperception process. Researchers such as Révész (1934) and most others regard it to be a result of "overlearned" stored memory content, i.e., the issue of

highly rigid constancy. The ever-changing, perpetually moving reality never completely conforms to those stored mental representations which are the results of a long process of learning. As a consequence, the reflection of the real physical world will appear entirely or partly deformed in cognition, since the clash between the appearance of the reality and the already stored mental gestalt will lead to triumph of the latter.

3. The *rectifying* tendency constitutes the sober, restrained side of the illusions. Thanks to this temperate trend, the individuals will become aware that they probably are subject to distortions of the real stimuli. This corrective tendency of the cognitive process is active beginning in early childhood though old age. Piaget (1937–1954) distinguished two classes of illusions according to the rectifying effects: (a) those in which the corrective trends are continually growing with age and (b) those in which the repairing activities are permanently diminishing with advancing age.

The above-described features of the illusion phenomenon have been known since the turn of the century, but, unfortunately, psychological and psychophysical research has not added much to the picture. All three tendencies seem to be *unconscious* phenomena, but at the same time they are *compulsory*, i.e., individuals are not able to escape from their influence. Thus, they represent an event of general psychological validity.

The laws and rules of the formation of illusions were elucidated in the domain of vision. Lipps as well as his followers studied the colorful and suggestive "landscape" of visual illusions and successively deducted the regularities of these perceptive misrepresentations by the detailed fundamental dissection of the optical "anomalities." Later on, the principles of the visual illusions were extended over the distortions of other modalities, such as audition, smell, and taste. The perception of the posture of the head and of the body and their movements constituted a separate line of research in which illusions were taken into consideration to the same extent as the visual ones. It was Révész (1956) who underlined the importance of the initiator of the analysis on the perception of locomotion describing the phenomena of vection, of opto- and audio-kinetic delusions. In our age of spaceflights, these human distortions acquire considerable importance.

I am firmly convinced that it is next to impossible that visceral perceptive phenomena are a category devoid of distortions, exempt from illusions. The above enumeration of the diverse modalities of sensory deformations was motivated by my test: to try to conceive an inquiry into the eventual hidden existence of visceral illusions. If we approach carefully the earlier as well as the recent literature, it appears as if some "functional" disturbances of given internal organs and systems with yet unknown etiology would not represent as much overt pathological processes but rather some kind of anomalies closer to illusions. First, IBS might possess some elements of sensory distortions discussed earlier in this chapter (see pp. 153–154). Further, the so-called "lump in the throat" (globus hystericus), gastroesophageal reflux disease (GERD), and a whole series of esophageal disorders regarded up to the present as motility disorders (e.g., achalasia, diffuse esophageal spasm, nutcracker esophagus, chest pain of unknown ethiology; see *Bradley & Richter*, 1996) might reflect to some extent sensory delusions not investigated as yet. Moreover, visceral hyperalgesia, allodynia, and other forms of visceral hypersensitivity described correctly in detail recently by Mayer and Gebhart (1994) may also have some elements of distorted perception, namely, illusions,especially since these authors underline the multifactorial etiology of some bowel disorders: in addition to the well-studied IBS, also nonulcer dyspepsia and noncardiac chest pain. Apparently, GI functional disorders may be the most conspicuous "nominees" for visceral illusions, but, of course, representatives of other pathological categories, such as cardiovascular disorders, cannot be excluded either. For example, it is high time to reinvestigate the thoroughly studied cardiac ischemic disorders from the point of view of cognitive distortions.

We must be fully aware that mere "empty" declarations or simple desires, like the above-mentioned ones, do not enable us to start an investigation on the existence of visceral illusions. Adequate methods are needed first, but still missing. If we advocate the principles of the validity of general laws of sense organs in the domain of *every* sensory system, we must find earlier or later the homologues or counterparts of the viscerosensory apparatus in this domain. For the time being we must be satisfied with the chances offered by some results obtained in the field of *haptic* (tactile) illusions. The mechano- and thermoreceptive activities of the dermal sense organs constitute in all probability those sensory functions that might be regarded as rather similar to visceral thermal or mechanical receptors and to their central representations (see p. 120).

I am quite convinced that future research in visceral illusions will start in several directions. One of these will probably be the experimental psychology of symptom reports as outlined in Chapter 12. All three tendencies (i.e., shaping, altering, and rectifying processes) of the distortions in the course of formation of illusions can be discovered in symptom psychology, but that is another story (details in Chapter 12).

In this modest essay I want to draw attention to the chances of visceral illusion research as a follow-up to the interrupted investigation of Révész (1928, 1934) in the domain of haptic illusions. Starting his exploration in the field of tactile agnosia or astereognosia, he switched soon to the problems of haptic distortions, which are in fact the combinations of tactile and motor misperceptions. He succeeded in proving some common rules of optic and haptic spatial distortions and even more: some special principles of the tactile–kinesthetic modality. Notwithstanding that some well-known peculiar haptic illusions (e.g., the so-called Aristotelian illusion: by rolling a small marble ball between our crossed index finger and middle finger we always have the feeling of two balls being rolled) have been known for thousands of years, Révész had accomplished an important, long-needed work. I enumerate here a few preconditions of the appearance and disappearance of haptic cognitive distortions assumed by this author:

1. Seizing the tactile stimulus in its integrity, i.e., grasping at once the whole object, instead of sweeping back and forth, or moving to and fro. In effect, this means the application of the Gestalt principle in the haptic field (Benussi, 1914).
2. Observing an optimal length of time for the formation of an illusion effect. It turned out that the optimal period of time is by no means a long interval; on the contrary, the cognitive haptic distortions become more obvious if the exposition period is short. The longer the exposition, the smaller the distortion.
3. Comparison of haptic stimuli inhibits the development of the illusions. The active exploration of the conditions and of the single elements and fragments of the objects exposed in order to feel and to touch them does not facilitate formation of the illusions. Meticulous exposure diminishes illusions.

> Révész succeeded in outlining and experimentally proving a number of additional conditions of the above type without the intention, however, of exhausting the topic. It is my conviction that the time has come to resume investigation in the above field and to start research on visceral illusions eventually on the same track.

Instead of applying artificial techniques with the aim of attaining a chronic, steady irritation of a visceral organ and recording the eventual changes in cognitive style of the subjects kept under observation, we chose irritable bowel syndrome (IBS) patients. IBS seemed to be an appropriate model of chronic impact of viscerosensory pathology on brain functions, including cognitive ones (Drossman et al., 1990). IBS seems to represent one (if not the only one) of the illnesses linked to brain processing of incoming information originating from the gut (Mei, 1990). The Manning,Thompson, Heaton, and Morris (1978) criteria of IBS separate from the framework of this syndrome those symptoms that are of organic, or structural, nature. Irrespective of whether specialists are in agreement or not about the pathogenesis and etiology of the syndrome, every report underlines the lowered sensory threshold of the gut of IBS patients (Cook, Van Eeden, & 1987; Meunier, 1990). Without going further into the analysis of the very nature of the disease, we regard it as a firm model of prolonged pathological sensory influence originating from a large visceral area (Mayer & Gebhart, 1994; Accarino, Azpiroz, & Malagelada, 1995). More detailed data of this investigation have been reported elsewhere (Fent et al., 1998).

The experiments were carried out on 31 adults of both sexes: 21 IBS patients and 10 healthy controls. The very essence of the series was the approximation of the minimal intestinal distention detection thresholds of the subjects following their division into spatial versus verbal cognitive strategy groups, and into left versus right hemisphere preferent subjects. First the cognitive paper-and-pencil tests were performed, followed by approximation of the CLEM test. This consisted of electrooculographic recordings and additional visual observations. These two psychological tests were followed by an assessment of the minimal detectable distention threshold of the sigmoid colon. The latter consisted of the repeated inflation of a rubber balloon inserted 35–40 cm into the colon with the aid of a computer-driven pneumatic system. Several forced-choice-type test inflations were carried out in which the verbal or spatial cognitive style subjects had to push buttons to answer questions appearing on the screen of a monitor in the isolated experimental room. This procedure of "tracking" mechanical gut stimuli by applying the signal detection strategy, enabled us to estimate the visceral perception threshold of IBS patients and to compare this value with the threshold of normal controls. Even more importantly, the preliminary screening of the subjects according to their cognitive strategies and to their preferred CLEMs (also a validated personality trait) rendered possible a comparison of intestinal perception performance, cognitive style, and hemispheric preference. The relations proved to be unequivocal although in some cases unexplainable.

It was found that distention thresholds in the healthy control subjects were significantly lower in verbals and higher in spatials. In IBS subjects these parameters were reversed: Gut perception thresholds were significantly higher in verbals and lower in spatials (Fig. 18). With regard to hemispheric preferents (thus habitual left or right eye movers), in control subjects the left hemisphere preferents had a significantly higher colonic perception threshold than the right hemisphere preferents. In the IBS group the tendency of threshold differences between right- and left-preferent patients was minimal.

A superficial survey of the above psychophysiological findings—the inverse relationship of cognitive style and of hemi-

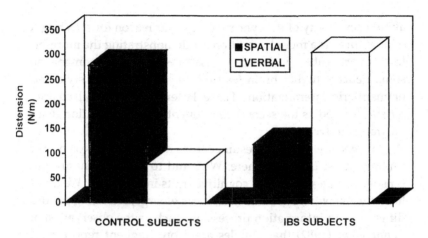

Figure 18. Colon distention threshold data (expressed in N/m) of the verbal and of the spatial subgroups in control and in IBS subjects according to the tracking procedure described in the text. The colon distention threshold is significantly higher in the spatial controls than in the verbal controls. It is reversed in the IBS patients: the threshold of the verbal patients is significantly higher than that of the spatials. From Fent *et al.* (1998).

spheric preference to colonic sensations in healthy and IBS subjects—fails to produce any integration under the umbrella of a single principle of visceral perception. If, however, we analyze somewhat more rigorously the given data, a possible common denominator might be revealed.

In a second look at the relatively small group of IBS patients, the correlation between colon sensitivity and some important, but subtle psychophysiological indices (spatial versus verbal information processing and hemispheric preference) proved to be inverted when compared with a relatively small group of healthy controls. The first component of this correlation, namely, the alteration of sensibility of the sigmoid colon in IBS, is well known from the literature, being the firm background of the six criteria of the disease described by Manning *et al.* (1978). This acknowledged altered sensitivity of the syndrome was our reason for selecting it in our study as a model condition for demonstrating the more-or-less covert, subtle influence of viscerosensory phenomena on some delicate higher brain features such as cognitive style and hemispheric lateralization. These latter psychological characteristics served as the second component of the correlation demonstrated above.

Consequently, the presumed common denominator of our findings must be sought here: Why and to what extent are gut sensory changes and brain cognitive traits interrelated? We don't have the answers, but some faint ideas emerge, reflecting gender differences in information processing, such as the observation of Pennebaker (1982) that females are more frequent reporters of physical symptoms than males. The tendencies are promising, and need to be reinforced by future studies.

Deficient Semiotics: An Obstacle to Visceral Cognition?

In the course of our experimentation on humans, seeking to approach and quantify the more-or-less covert visceral experience of our subjects, we had to apply several roundabout techniques, since the lack of verbal reportability rendered absolutely necessary such a circumvention. In Chapter 7, I described in detail four main indirect methods suited to replace direct verbal accounts. Originally such detours were suggested by Békésy (1947) and others with an aim different from ours, namely, to avoid verbal reportability, which always hides some subjective fluctuations. In contrast to this situation, our examination into the detectability of visceral changes highlighted the deficiency, or even the complete lack, of verbalization of these internal events. The very limited vocabulary of labeling visceral phenomena was a strong thread running through our studies. We concluded that the deficient semiotics may simply reflect that there is no need for humans in their normal everyday life to identify and to name mostly dim internal occurrences, except in emergency situations. As a typical sign of the very meager situation in "visceral semiotics," consider that Pennebaker (1982) reported an inventory of physical symptoms (Pennebaker Inventory of Limbic Languidness) consisting of 54 items, not more than one third of which refer to visceral processes (e.g., "lump in the throat," "racing heart"); the other two thirds reflect extero- and proprioceptive phenomena. Here I must make a slight digression: in contrast to the European–American one, the Asian–Oceanian cultural tradition, might be much more sensitive to observing internal changes and giving special attention to visceral phenomena, as exemplified by the ancient practice of the Indian Yogis. The significance of this rather anecdotal historical element should be scrupulously studied.

At the moment, it seems quite obvious that the deficient viscerosensory semiotics of our cultural heritage is the product of a very long history of the development of human languages (Trabant, 1996). In studying this evolution of literacy, beginning in the Paleolithic Age some 40,000 years ago, we can surmise that the anatomical and psychophysiological possibilities were always "at hand" for *Homo sapiens* to steadily transform nonreportable, thus nonconscious, visceral sensations into verbally reportable ones via learning. This means that nonconscious internal messages were permanently present necessarily influencing behavior, but their transition through conditioning into conscious, labeled perceptions proved to be unnecessary, thus redundant (except for the few urgency signals that have been mentioned). This lesson also reveals that in the cultural history of mankind, the activity of naming phenomena, objects, or concepts is a dynamic, fulminant, and steady process. Consider the verbalized world around us and how very different it is from one of some millennia, or even some centuries ago. Thus, the process of transforming nonverbalized visceral sensations into conscious perceptions by learning and identifying them through a "viscerosensory dictionary" is theoretically possible. In such a way, our knowledge about events occurring inside the body would enlarge substantially, increasing the "visceral cognition" of humans about themselves.

What theoretical or practical conclusions can be drawn from the above speculation? In principle, there are two alternative answers: (1) visceral education or (2) visceral oblivion!

1. Should experimental psychology or clinical neurophysiology aim at a special "visceral teaching program" so as to teach more and more people to perceive and label more and more as yet unperceived internal events? In our opinion, this strategy would considerably enlarge our cognitive maps, but at what price? The advanced ability to perceive large amounts of visceral phenomena may be beneficial for one group of people, who could keep under constant surveillance their internal processes, but harmful for another group of people developing pathological forced attention to visceral events, the roots of hypochondriasis (Pennebaker, 1982). Science is far from identifying the preliminary conditions and limitations of visceral perceptual learning. In all probability, personality factors are essential, but we are are again from constructing even an approximative consistent theory of viscerosensory personality traits.

2. Should clinical neuroscience and experimental psychology merely aim at the "indoors" continuation of carrying out high-level and serious research projects in order to elucidate the physiological and mental backgrounds and laws of visceral cognition, but strictly prohibiting the introduction of the results and the consequences of such "intramural" research into broader practice? We are convinced that this alternative is the right one at present. Much more scrupulous research and prudent ethical and

legal considerations are needed in order to resolve in the future the artificial, forced interference in the flow of a multimillennial evolution of semiotics.

In effect, if we admit the bifurcation of cognitive processes into a more ancient and diffuse protopathic segment and a more novel and well-delimited epicritic segment and if we attach to both of these segments a nonconscious, nonreportable as well as a conscious, reportable column, in this case visceral sensations and perceptions can be located simultaneously in all four compartments just enumerated (Fig. 19). These four conceptual categories form in an integrated way the rather articulated phenomenon regarded by us as "visceral cognition." Namely, some visceral messages, no doubt the majority, bear a rather protopathic character, and other signals a more-or-less epicritic feature. In the framework of both protopathic and epicritic segments one can situate visceral inputs that do not reach the level of reportability and others that, in an inborn, inherent, or learned way, prove to be verbally reportable and hence conscious. The wise acceptance of this natural compartmentalization has at present no alternative either from the point of view of brain sciences, or from the standpoint of ethics and jurisprudence.

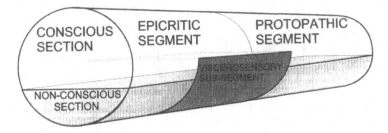

Figure 19. Schematic "cone of cognition," representing the viscerosensory subsegment situated between the protopathic and epicritic segments, on the border line between the nonconscious and conscious sections.

CHAPTER *12*

Visceral Perception and Symptom Report
An Epilogue

In the Preface I stated that when considering the cognitive aspects of visceroception, I stand somewhere halfway between "pure experimental" and "ecological" sensory physiology and psychology. This reflects my early acceptance of the fact that in addition to the physiologically rooted viscerosensory trend, represented by the present volume, a second, rather cognitive tendency has emerged, rooted in ecological and social psychology. The representative contemporary author of this novel direction, James W. Pennebaker (1982, 1985, 1995), has stated: "visceral perception does not occur in vacuo" (1985, p. 155). By this he meant that all individuals perceive and report physical symptoms and that these symptoms are always subject to distortions in each stage of perception. The distortions caused by already existing, stored sets, expectations and brain schemes will modify the "pure" percepts. This is why the researcher is steadily confronted with the dilemma: "laboratory" or "field" research in visceroception? In the Preface I asserted my "half-and-half" opinion. In the preceding chapters I tried to argue in favor of my point of view.

The fundamental starting assumptions of both "physiological" and "symptom-oriented" internal perception research happened to be identical: Bykov (1947) had formulated that the encoding of internal sensory information represents the same processes that have been elucidated by studying classical sense organs, i.e., the perception of external stimuli. This approach was literally reformulated by some authors of the "symptom-oriented" trend, e.g., Pennebaker (1982, p. 19). Incidentally, in this and similar "rediscoveries" by a given group of scientists of some facts and assumptions elucidated 30–40 years earlier by another, isolated team of researchers, I thought I saw the same "parallel history" (see pp. 19–25).

The history of the "symptom-oriented" research unfortunately reflects the past split between Eastern European and American tendencies focused on identical topics with similar approaches, although not taking notice of each other. Neither the pioneering paper of Cannon and Washburn (1912) on subjective symptom report of hunger following stomach contractions, nor the much later articles of Mandler *et al.* (1958), Stunkard and Koch (1964), and Stern *et al.* (1980) had aroused the interest of European, mostly Eastern European, physiologically oriented researchers working in the fields of visceral sensations and perceptions. All the more so since the "symptom-oriented" research people had turned toward cognitive tradition. It will suffice to mention the Schachter and Singer (1962) paper on cognitive labeling of emotions, that of Mechanic (1972) on labeling internal sensations of illness, and that of Leventhal (1980) and his group on parallel processing of the internal symptoms and their emotional aspects. There is no doubt that the inverse was also true: the "symptom-oriented" researchers did not count in general on data obtained earlier by the "experiment-driven" groups.

Consequently, we are witnessing today a peculiar situation in which dedicated scholars sometimes differ in their opinions due to their scientific education, philosophical outlook, methodological expertise, and so on. For example, consider the crucial term *symptom*. The entry in the *Oxford Student's Dictionary* (1988) under that headword states: "a change in the body's condition that is the sign (of illness): *symptoms of measles*." This short description fully corresponds to the meaning acquired in medical school as a student and very frequently used as such. Consequently, the "symptom" is an objectively *existing* element of the internal environment and the respective specialist (e.g., physician, chemist) is the appropriate person to specify it. The patient *is not* the right person to determine the existence or absence of the particular internal stimulus; he or she is entitled only to report on his or her *belief* as to the occurrence or the disappearance of the bodily sign. This is the point of view of medical people. In contrast, other scientists have a much broader definition of the term, including even subjective, distorted, or naive guesses, beliefs, and so on. Thus, "symptom-oriented" authors distinguish at least *two* classes of "symptom reporters": the subject and the "professional symptom decoder" (i.e., the physician or psychologist), both in equal measure. Sometimes the naive parent is also promoted to the rank of a reporter (Pennebaker, 1982). Such an "egalitarianism" of the three kinds of "symptom reporters" does not make analysis easy for the sober research scientist. But despite this terminological difference, symptom-oriented and experiment-oriented mentalities must and can find a common language when it comes to interpretations of their findings.

A much more substantial lack of mutual comprehension is found in the different approaches to the notion of "visceral perception" itself. I detailed in Parts I and II (pp. 3–8 and 13–16) my self-restraints and delimitations, and shall not revisit them here. Scientists working in our field of visceroception must regret that we are not close to each other with some symptom-oriented colleagues when it comes to defining and delimiting "visceral perception" and "symptom-perception." These are not synonyms at all. Symptom-oriented authors, regrettably, place an equality sign between radically different "physical symptoms" from finger temperature and pain to blood pressure. Whereas feelings of heat, cold, or pain originating from the cutaneous layers of the extremities are physiologically far from being "internal" sensations, guesses as to the arterial pressure exerted on the wall of blood vessels are typical visceral sensations. When analyzing internal symptoms one can hardly mix the two completely different sensory categories. Consider a fictional situation in which we intermingle all classical senses (from vision to tactile sensitivity) and consequently we analyze their symptoms under a unified "umbrella," pretending that we are opening a peculiar integrated "sense black box." Such a confused procedure would be inconceivable for a physiologist. Of course, common laws and principles of all sense organs do exist and they must be revealed. Nonetheless, the rules of each sense apparatus should be elucidated separately, including the symptoms that they produce. In this way, we cannot put "physical symptoms" into a single, unified category from nasal congestion through heart-rate approximation up to blood sugar estimation, because these are completely different entities for physiology, obeying distinct rules and laws. Before searching for common denominators among them (and we should not doubt the existence of common features), we are obliged to delimit and characterize the symptoms separately, one after the other, in order to be aware of the problems requiring formulation of appropriate answers. Just such a delimitation and characterization was the aim of the different chapters of this book. For the superficial reader, it may appear that I did not discover enough justification for the symptom-oriented principles. Not in the least: I am quite convinced that the symptom-oriented trend is a very important contribution to viscerosensory research, just from the cognitive point of view. Our neurophysiologically rooted endeavors and symptom-oriented efforts successfully supplement each other, as stated in the Preface.

The advantages of the symptom-report-based cognitive direction are obvious for the experiment-oriented researcher. These include, among others:

1. Placing cognitive brain *schemes* into the forefront. We hold, without reservation, that the representations in the brain reflecting the distorted reality are the prime movers of symptom reports.
2. Hence, the emphasis placed on the *distortions* caused by sets, expectations, and beliefs stored in the memory of the subjects (e.g., the causes of placebo effects).
3. The stress laid on *social* psychological aspects of expectations and naive beliefs deeply influencing distorted reports of internal symptoms.
4. Drawing the attention of clinical medicine to the importance of internal reports as *alarming signals* that may be lifesaving (e.g., hypoglycemia).

The drawbacks of the symptom-oriented principles were outlined above, and the experiment-oriented researcher will be unable to evaluate some general conclusions drawn from symptom reports. After all, a considerable uneasiness will accompany the assessment of some results obtained via common research paradigms, e.g., between blood pressure reports and blood sugar evaluations, since the physiological mechanisms of these two kinds of messages are completely different. In our opinion, only a consideration of both the detailed physiological background *and* the cognitive aspects of a given symptom evaluation can lead to valid results.

Among misunderstandings that still remain between physiologically oriented and some symptom report-prone authors, I must mention the divergent approaches of the voluntarily not susceptible, i.e., automatic and unintentional, homeostatic regulations. There is no doubt about the existence of reliably functioning autonomic regulations, such as isoglycemia, isohydria, isovolemia, and isosmosis. As far as is known, such autonomic balances are not subject to *voluntary* corrections or switches from autonomic (vegetative) nervous influences or volitional hormonal (humoral) interventions. Consider the following quote from an important article: "When we hold our breath for several seconds, the unpleasant sensations that we begin to experience usually aid us in our ultimate decision to recommence inhaling and exhaling" (Pennebaker *et al.*, 1985). This sentence suggests that the subject decides whether to breathe or not. The reality is totally different: the individual is not capable of choosing to inhale or not to inhale. If the hypercapnia (elevation of CO_2 in the arterial blood) reaches a certain critical value, the inspiration neurons in the medulla, which regulate breathing and are under the control of blood gases, emit impulses of inhalation. There is no way to escape from this control.The compulsory command of the CO_2-driven bulbar respiratory neurons overcomes any volitional act regardless of how intensive it might be. There are a number of well-stabilized mechanisms that automatically make adjustments of a given function (e.g., blood pressure, blood pH, blood glucose) to its optimal set point. Any deflection from the adjusted set point automatically triggers the innate processes for restoration of the optimum value.

A "roundabout" way may be employed to influence these automatic mechanisms. Such an indirect possibility makes use of the *somatic motor* apparatus (mostly in a conscious from), in order to intervene in the automatic adjustment. Blood glucose and pH can be modified temporarily by food, fluid, and drug intake, blood pressure by medication and special manipulations (e.g., Valsalva maneuver), and so on. However, in most cases, these external interventions only temporarily affect the firmly organized inherent homeostatic set points. The "roundabout" approach is, in essence, nothing but the *somatic mediation* of visceral afferent and efferent effects amply discussed in this book (see pp. 15, 100).

The dominant nature of these innate, persistent and conservative homeostatic regulations and the permanent prevalence of their physiological constant values, which function mostly in a nonconscious way and which form the firm basis of the normal life of all organisms, must not be forgotten. Neglect of this basic principle may lead to a peculiar "psychological voluntarism," i.e., to the erroneous view that most, if not all, visceral phenomena can be changed by focusing attention, by conditioning, and the like. Such "voluntarism" can be found in some psychoanalytically oriented theories and practices advocating the healing power of bringing to light (i.e., to consciousness) nonconscious automatisms. Such explorations, according to their adherents, render some autonomic phenomena accessible to deliberate manipulations.

Classical physiological data unequivocally demonstrate that as far as the viscerosensory input is concerned, it forms everywhere the afferent branch of the above-described nonconscious innate homeostatic loops. If necessary for survival, it forces its way through to consciousness, as we have seen for emergency situations modeled in our visceroceptive learning experiments. Otherwise, most visceral messages remain in the nonconscious domain. And in all probability they should remain there, serving before all the rigid autonomic regulations of vitally indispensable homeostasis. Consequently, instead of emerging into consciousness by constraint, the majority of these autonomic control mechanisms should remain nonconscious. Rather than striving after steady remembrance, on the contrary, an effort for oblivion, for neglect of internal processes should guide normal human behavior. In Chapter 11 I emphasized that the long process of transforming nonverbalized visceral sensations into conscious perceptions by learning and of identifying them through the creation of a peculiar "viscerosensory vocabulary" is *theoretically* possible but practically unnecessary, and even, apparently, harmful. Psychophysiology should not aim at a special "viscerosensory training program." Human visceral perception should remain at the doorsteps of cognition!

PART V

Appendixes

The following three appendixes are from earlier published original texts relevant to the topic of this volume. Appendix I is an excerpt from a previous monograph written by the author in 1967 and amply cited in this volume. It is intended to clarify the view of the author on consciousness. Appendixes II and III, an earlier book chapter by W. E. Whitehead (1983) and a recent paper by Neal E. Miller (1992), respectively, may also enrich the information contained in this volume, since the way of thinking of these scholars is very close to that of the author. The excerpts published here include their original bibliographies; consequently; the reoccurence of some citations in the References chapter of this volume could not be avoided.

APPENDIX *I*

Interoception and Consciousness

In the foregoing chapters the material presented has been obtained by animal experiments. For obvious reasons, behaviour research, like other disciplines of neurobiology, cannot be conducted without zoological experimental objects, though the final aim of all investigations on higher nervous activity is to understand the laws of human mental functions. Thus, also the above-described experimental results help to approach human interoception.

The sixty years of behaviour research have been an unremitting endeavour to throw light on the laws governing mental processes, and the data derived from animal experiments concerning higher nervous activity have been repeatedly confirmed in humans, too. There is, however, a lack of reliable and comprehensive original data about interoception in man, and especially about its connexion with behaviour. When attempting to find an explanation for the lack of such data in the literature, one must return to the argument already mentioned (Chapter I, p. 3), that impulses arriving from the visceral field do not lead to subjective sensation,

From G. Ádám: *Interoception and behaviour.* Akadémiai Kiadó, Budapest, 1967.

171

hence, they fail to reach consciousness. In addition, they are accessible by objective methods only exceptionally.

The question of consciousness gives rise to a number of problems. When interpreting our experimental results and the corresponding data of the literature it has been emphasized that learned processes of both somatic and visceral origin are governed by the same laws. We believe that this assumption is justifiable as far as animals are concerned. However, it cannot be applied automatically to humans. The problem of consciousness is the dividing point between animal and human research on the relation of interoception and behaviour. Patterns of behaviour controlled by exteroceptive, and in part also by proprioceptive stimuli, are mostly conscious or can be brought into consciousness. This cannot be said of interoceptive impulses, especially when speaking about their influence upon higher nervous activity.

Before going into a detailed discussion of the relation of interoception to consciousness in view of our own experimental results, a brief review of the present knowledge on conscious and unconscious psychic functions will be given on the basis of contemporary neurophysiological and psychological literature.

Some Remarks on Unconscious Mental Processes

The manner of treating our subject in this Chapter will be somewhat different from that used hitherto, when we restricted ourselves to the description of our experimental results and their strictly physiological interpretation. Here, while discussing consciousness from a physiological point of view, problems will arise that reach beyond the physiological aspects of behaviour and enter the realm of psychology.

Undoubtedly, human observation has distinguished two categories of afferent nervous mechanisms in the form of conscious and unconscious components of reflexes, and to throw light on the essential properties of these mechanisms is a basic task of neurophysiological research. The concepts of the conscious and unconscious have been explained in many ways by philosophers, psychologists, anthropologists, sociologists and psychiatrists in the course of the past decades. Only the physiological aspects of this question will be taken into consideration here. Physiologists have not been able to come to a uniform conclusion either concerning the definition of conscious and unconscious; this is clearly reflected in the material of various symposia held in the United States between 1950 and 1954 and published by Abramson (1950–54), and in the debates on the philosophical aspects of higher nervous activity and psychology, which were going on in the Soviet Union (Bassin 1963).

It is common knowledge that, when being awake, the activity level of higher nervous centres increases, which is manifested by a lowering of the threshold to afferent input. As already discussed (Chapter III, p. 53), the brain stem reticular substance plays a prominent part in this phenomenon.

Wakefulness is a precondition of, but not identical with the physiological concept of consciousness. The absence of waking renders any perception or cognizance impossible. On the other hand, in the state of wakefulness, we become aware of some afferent impulses (mostly exteroceptive ones), and do not know of others (mostly interoceptive ones), although on the basis of our experiments it is evident that also interoceptive input reaches the higher centres, moreover, it may activate the reticular formation. It seems likely that arousal is a prerequisite of, but does not account for consciousness—as it is believed by some authors relying on the hypothesis of *centrencephalon* (Penfield, 1938).

According to the conditioned reflex theory, consciousness means that impulses entering as primary signals assume a secondary signalizing character (Kardos 1957). External input is not only perceived, but at the same time *known of*, as it is clearly indicated by the Latin word *conscientia*. Thus, this theory regards the bringing of an impulse into consciousness as the synchronous appearance of the concrete primary, and the abstract secondary, signal in the higher nervous centres. This conception is similar to the old psychological definition according to which consciousness is the entirety of all sensations and psychic phenomena present in the brain at a given time. In view of this approach, consciousness involves the synchronous activity of several functional entities of the nervous system, presumably cortical and subcortical structures. It is also possible that these structures, while determining consciousness, constitute a functional system. Maybe, Leontyev (1959) was right, when he commented on the ideas of N.A. Bernstein, as follows: "Observations with contemporary methods indicate that, from a physiological point of view, every activity may be defined as a dynamic functional system that is governed by the varying and complex signals arriving from the external and internal environment. These signals reach the various nervous centres, among others the proprioceptive centre; in these greatly interdependent centres the signals are synthetized. Activity is characterized, neurologically, by the participation of different nervous centres. Activity becomes realized at different levels of the nervous system, with the participation of different structures. These levels are, however, not equally important. One of the structures predominates, while the others form the background or basis (Bernstein defined them as "basic levels"). Bernstein has emphasized the remarkable fact that of the signals belonging to the sphere of perception always the decisive ones, those of the highest rank, become conscious. Thus, the recognized conscious content governs the activities of various structures" [author's translation from the Russian original].

If this hypothesis is accepted as a starting point, the following questions immediately arise: why do interoceptive impulses remain at the unconscious level, why do we not become aware of them, and are they able to leave the "background" and enter consciousness? Attempts will be made to answer these questions in view of our experimental results. Let us first make a few remarks about the unconscious, the level of functional organization up to which most of the interoceptive impulses arrive.

We have chosen a motto by Freud to this chapter although we cannot agree with his neuropsychiatrical and philosophical views. Nevertheless, we wish to pay tribute to his role in arousing the interest of experimenters and clinicians in unconscious mental processes.

It would be far beyond the scope of this work to discuss and criticize the Freudian theory, and the various neo-Freudian ideas. The influence of Freud has been immense and although his ideas have never been physiologically verified and are mostly antiquated, one cannot disregard a theory which has played such a prominent part in determining the development of neuropsychiatry and which was, after all, the product of an ingenious personality. Here only the Freudian theory on consciousness will be reviewed concerning interoception.

Freud has stated clearly and unambiguously that behaviour is determined not only by environmental and social factors, and is governed not only by conscious processes, but also by processes occurring in the sphere of mental functions which he called unconscious. This is the basic issue of his conception and this is how far—and only that far—we completely agree with him. A series of arguments presented in connexion with the results of our animal experiments pointed to the considerable influence and control of visceral afferent impacts on behaviour. The visceral afferentation studied in our experiments is, without doubt, unconscious. We are of the opinion that interoceptive information, together with humoral-hormonal and proprioceptive influences, constitute the main source of impulses determining the unconscious sphere of behaviour. At this point the course of our argument leaves the Freudian line.

The neurophysiologist cannot call in question the existence of unconscious psychic processes; the experimental data to be reviewed in this Chapter demonstrate that unconscious mental phenomena, a concept which, for a long time, has been monopolized by the psychoanalytic school, are based on well-defined physiological mechanisms. Thus, the question today is not whether unconscious psychic activity is a reality, but what it essentially is, and what is its mechanism.

Freud distinguished preconscious (*Vorbewusstsein*) and unconscious (*Unbewusstsein*) processes. The former is easily converted into conscious, while the latter is not, or only with difficulty. Our experimental work is concerned first of all with the first category. Freud wrote: "The unconscious system may therefore be compared to a large ante-room, in which the various mental excitations are crowding upon one another, like individual beings. Adjoining this is a second, smaller apartment, a sort of reception room, in which consciousness resides."

Apart from the vulgar metaphor and the unscientific presentation, Freud seems to have foreseen the elements of a very important mechanism. Nevertheless, in this definition no mention has been made yet about what he believed to be the contents of the preconscious phase, about his view that both the unconscious and preconscious processes are formed in early childhood. According to Freud, the psychic life after puberty has almost no history.

Freud maintained that the content of the unconscious phases is only sexual and self-preservative in character, and the individual is unable to adapt itself to the biological and social environment owing to the unmanageable and uncontrollable unconscious, the inherited, mystical and primordial: *das Es*, which the consciousness is unable to govern. According to Freud, consciousness and unconsciousness are two opposing poles. The neurophysiologist feels the whole sequence of ideas to be false. Especially the psychoanalytic theory, based on this theory of instincts, strikes one as unscientific: the overestimation and overcommenting of sexual and self preservative instincts, and the constrained interpretation of errors, dreams, the concept of repression and, finally, the employment of absurd symbols and mythological analogies.

The criterium of Freudian theory is the interpretation of the content of the unconscious system. It seems absurd to us to restrict the unconscious to several instinctive mechanisms, even if acknowledging the great importance of these instincts. Contemporary neurophysiology has collected an immense amount of data on the mechanism of the almost entirely mesodiencephalic instinctive and emotional functions which play a prominent part in determining behaviour. Of the numerous observations let us only mention the work of Lissák and his school (Lissák 1958; Lissák and Endrőczi 1965; Grastyán 1958). Clearly, most of these processes in man are unconscious, though not in the Freudian sense, for they do not *ab ovo* restrain behaviour and are not repressed counterparts of the rational conscious system. Even though its mechanism is not yet well understood, instinctive drive might in many cases act as a synergist of conscious, socially determined, or even learned processes. Naturally, in certain cases it might act as their antagonist. Nevertheless, it is a fundamental pillar, the basis of complex learned processes; and one of the most important afferent systems related to the instinctive sphere is the interoceptive system. In agreement with other critics, we appreciate Freud the ingenious empiricist and phenomenologist but reject his theory on instincts, which is neurophysiologically unfounded. Undoubtedly, Freud's empiricism has placed the question of the unconscious in the focus of interest, which is his merit even if he drew exaggerated conclusions regarding the content of the unconscious sphere. The problem is inevitably encountered by the neurophysiologists following the Pavlovian theory, especially since the categories of conscious and unconscious are, oddly enough, completely absent from the conditioned reflex theory. Without understanding these categories, it is impossible to study the function and significance of the interoceptive system in man.

The Physiological Aspects of Human Interoception: Do We Return to the James–Lange Theory?

Surveying the immense literature on the complex problem of consciousness, we have come to the conclusion that the development of human consciousness is the most reasonably explained by the materialistic theory according to which consciousness is a product of man's social existence, and develops in connection with active human labour. From the physiological point of view, the development of consciousness, thus, depends entirely on exteroceptive impulses, for both social life and work involve the analysis and synthesis by the central nervous system of external inputs. What is then the role of interoception in human psychical processes, if there is any?

In our opinion, interoception in man might have three main functions:

1. Interoceptive impulses control the normal functioning of organs and systems from which they arise. This is essentially a feed-back servo-mechanism which ensures the maintenance of the constancy of the internal milieu and the homeostasis of the organism. This control is not restricted to the organ from which the afferent impulse arises, but involves other organs or organ systems as well (viscero-visceral reflexes); moreover, the efferent branch of the reflex might be purely somatic (viscero-somatic reflexes). This function of the interoceptive system is well known to classical physiology (cf. Chapter I, pp. 15, 18).

2. Interoceptive impulses inform the higher centres about conditions which necessitate active operant responses. This kind of emergency information which allows adaptation to the external environment includes such conditions as hunger, thirst and the excretion of waste matters.

When fulfilling this second task, interoceptive activity may be on the same level as exteroceptive impulses, and may even become conscious. As already discussed, the transmission of stimuli concerning micturition and defecation is an important task of the interoceptive system; these impulses are brought into consciousness in the early phases of ontogenesis by conditioned reflexes. These signals are important in controlling also conscious psychical functions and behaviour.

3. In view of our experimental data we are inclined to suggest that, besides the above two functions (control of organ functions and signalization of conscious requisite conditions), most interoceptive inputs have a part, so to say, somewhere between the two, i.e., they have an intermediate function. Such impulses not only exert a feedback control but explicitly influence behaviour, without giving rise to subjective sensations, i.e., without entering consciousness. It has been repeatedly observed in our animal and human experiments that associative functions originate from the visceral receptor field, which are not directly related to the external environment and operant activities, still they exist and have an effect on behaviour, although they remain fully unconscious. To which category do these associative impulses belong that do not determine human activity? What is the function of this unconscious visceral information? Our hypothesis is that they might play a role in determining the emotional state of man.

As it is known, James (1884) in America and Lange (1905) in Denmark were the first, in 1884, to give, independently of each other, a scientific definition of emotion. According to them, emotion is not a primary condition but the reflection in the higher nervous system of the state of the visceral sphere. There are some differences between the theories of Lange and James: Lange, e.g., attributed a prominent part to the cardiovascular system. Nevertheless, they both assume that the affective features of psychical activity are primarily determined by visceral inputs. They believe that impacts from the external environment, with the mediation of the cerebral cortex, cause changes in the function of the visceral organs, which, in turn, being re-transmitted to the central nervous system give rise to emotional expression.

The theory of James and Lange has been overshadowed, owing to the rapid development in other field of physiology and to the lack of interest in interoception. Many respectful physiologists, e.g., Cannon (1927, 1931) in the nineteen-thirties, having in mind the role of subcortical structures, sharply criticized this theory. Interestingly enough, even the psychoanalytic school rejected the James-Lange theory. Freud wrote in his book *A General Introduction to Psychoanalysis* (p. 403): "What psychology has to say about affects—the James-Lange theory, for instance—is utterly incomprehensible to us psychoanalysts and impossible for us to discuss."

How much do we know about the physiological mechanisms of emotion? Since the work of Darwin (1872) who analysed the role of mimetic muscles in the evolution of emotion, workers of almost every biological and physiological school have dealt with this even hitherto unknown mechanism. The data revealed probably will all contribute to the understanding of the complex organization of emotional behaviour, constituting particular elements of the entire mechanism. Such theories were, e.g., Cannon's (1931) thalamocortical conception, or the views concerning the diffuse reticular system (Lindsley 1951; Magoun 1958) and the limbic system (Papez 1937; Klüver and Bucy 1939).

While substantial evidence is available concerning the vegetative responses resulting from emotional states (Dunbar 1954), visceral events preceding affective processes have been dealt with to a lesser extent since James and Lange. Lissák (1958), while emphasizing the importance of the endocrine system in determining emotion, pointed out that, in view of the observations of Bykov (1947), the role played by the autonomic afferent nervous system must be taken into consideration.

Relying on our experimental data we presume that interoceptive impulses constitute an important afferent channel to cortical, limbic and mesencephalic structures governing emotional responses. The visceral signal seems to influence behaviour considerably both in man and animals, even though they become conscious in man only occasionally. Of course, it is impossible at present to assess the extent of this interoceptive influence upon emotion and behaviour. As our hypothesis has not been experimentally proved we do not wish to draw far-reaching conclusions and not in the least are we inclined to belong to the group of investigators of whom Brady (1960) rightly said: "In probably no other domain of physiological science has so little empirical data provided the occasion for so much theoretical speculation as in the general area of the 'emotions.'" We certainly need working hypotheses when trying to interpret the results of our animal and human experiments even if they must be modified or abandoned in the future.

In summarizing, we tend to believe that in man the majority of interoceptive impulses influence behaviour without, however, causing any subjective sensation. Probably future discoveries will rehabilitate the old, and at present thought of as antiquated, theory of James and Lange on the origin of emotions. The sphere of emotions might be influenced, besides other impacts, by visceral afferent impulses, or at least interoception might constitute one of the most important sources of information determining unconscious psychical functions. This involves not only unconditioned visceral afferent impulses, but also learned, conditioned interoceptive reactions. It seems likely that temporary connexions initiated by visceral receptors and affecting both vegetative and somatic functions are being continuously established and extinguished, while never becoming conscious. On the basis of our experimental data we suppose that the unconscious interoceptive sphere, too, has a "memory," i.e., an ability to retain experience, which helps adaptation to changes in the environment. These conditioned reflexes are similar to those elaborated by us in animals (rats, cats, dogs and monkeys) and humans and are mainly classified as viscero-visceral, though many are viscero-somatic.

In addition to the development of interoceptive conditioned reflexes, there exists the possibility of bringing some unconscious visceral afferent processes into consciousness by the way of conditioning, i.e., by associating them with consciously perceived, mostly verbal, exteroceptive stimuli.

The question might now arise as to whether the latter process of visceral impulses entering consciousness actually occurs in conditions of normal life. It can be assumed that the interoceptive components of functions important for the individual (hunger, thirst) and socially (micturition, defecation) become conditioned in early childhood with exteroceptive stimuli, and the reinforcement of impulses other than these would constitute too great a stress for higher nervous centres; in other words, to bring into consciousness such internal processes would be pathological.

When the patient suffering from heart disease "feels" the least decrease in the blood supply of the heart, he actually undergoes a long process of conditioning, the result of which is that, after several months of the disease, he becomes conscious of minor degrees of hypoxia. The basic prerequisite of the normal functioning of the organism seems to be that interoceptive impulses should remain unconscious.

Interoceptive conditioning in man is only a means of revealing the relation of visceral afferentation to behavioural reactions. In exceptional cases it might also be of therapeutic use, e.g., in nocturnal enuresis.

In general, our opinion about conditioning and bringing into consciousness of visceral afferent impulses is similar to that about the Freudian psychoanalytic therapy. In certain cases it might be possible that, for therapeutic purposes, unconscious instinctive processes should enter a conceptual or emotional system, i.e., are brought into consciousness by verbal stimuli, but such a treatment inevitably creates complexes, leading to neurosis. In most of the cases repression into the unconscious, hence oblivion, is a far better therapy.

The aim of research work on interoception cannot be to increase the conscious realization of visceral impacts, but to emphasize that man is healthy as long as visceral stimuli and the conditioned reflexes based on them remain unconscious.

On the other hand, it is necessary to improve our knowledge concerning the role played by interoception in determining and controlling, behaviour. It has been repeatedly underlined that the final aim of neurophysiological and behaviour research is to elucidate the human psychical functions. This aim cannot be attained without learning the role of the interoceptive system. It has been our endeavour to contribute to this important objective by the experimental work presented here.

References

Abramson, H. A. (1950–54). *Problems of consciousness*. Macy, New York.

Bassin, F. V. (1963). Soznanye i "bessoznatelnoe. " In *Philosophskye Voprossy Physiologii Vysshei Nervnoi Deyatelnosti i Psychologii*. Izd. An. USSR. Moscow.

Brady, J. V. (1960). Emotional behavior. In J. Field (ed.), *Handbook of physiology. Neurophysiology* (Vol. 3, pp. 1529–1552). Washington, DC: American Physiology Society.

Bykov, K. M. (1947). *Kora golovnovo mozga i vnutrennie organy*. Moscow: Medgiz.

Cannon, W. B. (1927). The James-Lange theory of emotions. A critical examination and an alternative theory. *Amer. J. Physiol., 39*, 106.

Cannon, W. B. (1931). Again the James-Lange and the thalamic theories of emotion. *Psychol. Rev., 38*, 281.

Darwin, C. (1872). *The expression of the emotions in man and animals*. London: John Murray.

Dunbar, H. F. (1954). *Emotions and bodily changes* (4th ed.). New York: Columbia.

Freud, S. (1960). *A general introduction to psychoanalysis.* New York: Washington Square Press.

Grastyán, E., Lissák, K., Kékesi, F., Szabó, J., & Vereby, I. (1958). Beiträge zur Physiologie des Hippocampus. *Physiol. Bohemoslov., 7*, 9.

James, W. (1884). What is an emotion? *Mind IX.*

Kardos, L. (1957). *A lélektan alapproblémái és a pavlovi kutatások* (Basic problems of psychology and the Pavlovian research). Budapest: Akadémiai Kiadó.

Klüvar, H., Búcy, P. C. (1939). Preliminary analysis of functions of the temporal lobes in monkeys. *Arch. Neurol. Psychiatr. (Chic.), 42*, 979–980.

Lange, C. G. (1905). *Les émotions. Étude psycho-physiologique* (2nd ed.). Paris: Félix Alcan.

Leontyev, A. N. (1959). *Problems of the evolution of the mind* [in Russian]. Moscow: Publishing House of the Academy of the USSR.

Lindsley, D. B. (1951). Emotion. In S. S. Stevens (Ed.), *Handbook of experimental psychology.* New York: Wiley.

Lissák, K. (1958). A magatartás kutatás néhány új problémája (Some recent problems of the research on behaviour). *Magy. Tud. Akad. Biol. Orv. Tud. Oszt. Közl., 9*, 397.

Lissák, K., & Endrõczi, E. (1965). *Neuroendocrine control of adaptation.* Budapest: Akadémiai Kiadó.

Magoun, H. W. (1958). *The waking brain.* Thomas, Springfield, Ill.

Papez, J. W. (1937). A proposed mechanism of emotion. *Arch. Neurol. Psychiatr. (Chic.), 38*, 725–732.

Penfield, W. (1938). The cerebral cortex in man. I. The cerebral cortex and consciousness. *Arch. Neurol. Psychiatry, 40*, 417.

APPENDIX *II*

Interoception
Awareness of Sensations Arising in the Gastrointestinal Tract

1. Introduction

A surprisingly large amount of sensory information comes to the central nervous system from the gut. There are more afferent fibers than efferent fibers in the extrinsic nerves which supply the gastrointestinal tract. Leek (1972) estimates that 80%–90% of fibers in the vagus (parasympathetic) nerves are afferent, more than 50% of fibers in the splanchnic (sympathetic) nerves are afferent, and approximately 30% of the fibers in the pelvic (parasympathetic) nerves are afferent.

The purpose of this chapter is to examine the ways in which this sensory information may influence behavior. The emphasis of the chapter will be on sensory information which reaches or has the potential for reaching subjective awareness. Subjective awareness is defined by verbal behavior (or overt skeletal muscle responses rendered equivalent to verbal responses by instructions) indicative of the accurate discrimination of gastrointestinal stim-

From William E. Whitehead in: *Psychophysiology of the gastrointestinal tract. Experimental and clinical applications.* Edited by Rupert Hölzl and William E. Whitehead. Plenum Press, New York, 1983.

uli which are either produced by the experimenter or, in the case of naturally occurring physiologic events, objectively measured by the experimenter.

Only a small portion of the sensory information which reaches the brain from the gut is available to awareness. This is not a matter of the more intense stimuli being perceived; rather, some types of sensations appear to be selectively represented in awareness.

The best general study of sensory awareness in the alimentary tract was published at the beginning of the century (Hertz, 1911). Hertz used the same investigative techniques which are employed currently with human subjects, namely, the introduction of fluids, balloons, and rods into the gut by mouth, by rectum, or through a gastrostomy, ileostomy, or colostomy. He concluded that the alimentary tract is insensitive to touch from the pharynx to the anal canal, but that touch is appreciated in the anal canal. Distension (stretching) is appreciated throughout the alimentary canal and is interpreted differently in different locations: In the esophagus, distension produces a sensation of fullness, and the subject can accurately point to the location of the balloon. Hertz believed that distension of the stomach produced a sensation of repletion or satiety but that contractions of an empty stomach were interpreted as hunger. Distension of the small or large bowel was felt as fullness and was often attributed to gas. Subjects could not localize the site of the intestinal stimulus. Distension of the rectum produced an urge to defecate. Hertz asserted that overdistension was the only source of pain originating in the gastrointestinal tract.

Hertz investigated other stimuli as well. He found that hot and cold stimuli were perceived in the esophagus down to the gastroesophageal sphincter and in the anal canal. Hertz felt that the evidence for perception of temperature in the colon was equivocal. Acids were not felt when instilled into the stomach or esophagus, but alcohol produced a sensation of warmth or burning when introduced into the stomach. In concentrations of 25%, alcohol also caused a burning sensation in the anal canal, and in concentrations of 50%–90% alcohol produced a sensation of heat in the colon. The anal canal, but not the rectum, was found by Hertz to be sensitive to stimulation by glycerine.

As evidence of the selectivity of perception in the alimentary tract Hertz was able to cite the experience of performing abdominal surgery without anesthesia—a practice more common at the turn of the century than presently. He reported that "the normal stomach, small intestine, colon, and appendix could be touched with cold or hot objects, burnt with a caustic, clipped with forceps, or cut with a knife without producing any sensation" (Hertz, 1911, p. 43). As further evidence of selectivity, Iggo (1957) has shown that there are vagal fibers which respond to acids, alkalies, and touch in the stomach, although these stimuli are not subjectively discriminated.

Hertz (1911) noted at the end of his excellent book that he had observed individual differences in the ability of his subjects to discriminate various stimuli. He found differences both in the threshold amount of intestinal distension required to produce a subjective sensation and differences in whether a thermal stimulus in the colon was perceived at all. Hertz suggested that some form of learning, or sensitization by "neurasthenia" and anemia, might account for such differences. However, experimental methods were not available at that time which would have enabled him to investigate these hypotheses. The next section describes the developments in investigative technique which have enabled the field of visceral perception to advance since the time of Hertz.

2. Methods of Investigating Visceral Perception

2.1. Method of Limits

In studying perception, it is useful to know not only whether a subject can perceive a stimulus, but also how intense the stimulus must be before it is perceived. This threshold is often estimated by progressively increasing the intensity of the stimulus until the subject reports that he perceives it and/or by progressively decreasing stimulus intensity until the subject reports that he can no longer detect it. This procedure, called the method of limits, has a serious limitation, however. It is now known that perceptual judgments are influenced by some non-perceptual variables which are collectively called response bias. An example of response bias would be the tendency of some subjects not to say they see a stimulus until they are absolutely certain because they wish to be seen as conservative, or the tendency of subjects not to report a painful stimulus until it is unbearable because they wish to be seen as strong. Other factors can shift the apparent threshold in the opposite direction; for example, the hunter who shoots at anything that moves because there is a high payoff for a hit and relatively little cost to a "false alarm."

2.2. Signal Detection Analysis

The method of limits does not permit actual perceptual sensitivity to be separated from response bias. However, there are two psychophysical procedures which do permit this separation. The first is based on the theory of signal detection (Swets, 1973). It involves presenting a large number of trials (200–500 trials) on each of which the subject is asked to judge whether or not the stimulus was presented. By examining the ratio of hits to misses and the ratio of false alarms to correct rejection (i.e., saying "no" when the stimulus was not presented), it is possible to obtain independent estimates of perceptual sensitivity and response bias. Stunkard and Fox (1971) and Whitehead and Drescher (1980) needed six experimental sessions to obtain 200 trials on a stomach contraction perception test.

2.3. Forced Choice Procedure

An alternative method of estimating perceptual sensitivity which requires fewer trials (approximately 20) is the forced choice procedure (Tanner & Swets, 1954). This involves always presenting the subject with a pair of trials and asking the subject to indicate whether the stimulus was presented in the first or second trial. The subject is told to guess if he is not sure. The stimulus is always presented in one of the two trials. This procedure is insensitive to most sources of response bias, although it will be affected by a strong preference for saying first or second and by a refusal to "guess." The chief limitation of the procedure is that very young children or cognitively impaired adults do not understand the instructions. Whitehead, Engel, and Schuster (1980) used this technique to assess awareness of pressure stimuli in the colon.

2.4. Confounding of Perception and Control

When the goal of an experiment is to assess the subject's perception of a naturally occurring physiologic response such as a stomach contraction rather than his perception of an artificial stimulus such as a balloon inflation, an additional problem arises: One must be able to distinguish between the ability of the subject to voluntarily emit or alter the response and his ability to discriminate occurrence of the response. The importance of this distinction is illustrated by the literature on the discrimination of one's own heart rate. Brener and Jones (1974) developed a procedure for testing heart rate perception by asking the subject to judge whether a sequence of vibratory stimuli were triggered by the R-wave of the EKG or by a machine which produced a train of pulses at a frequency equal to the subject's average heart rate. However, Ross and Brener (1981) subsequently discovered that subjects solved this task by taking a deep breath and observing whether or not this produced a change in the pattern of stimuli. Subjects are less knowledgeable about how to voluntarily control most gastrointestinal responses. However, since these perception tests are often done in the context of biofeedback experiments, one must be careful to make the test of discrimination independent of the subject's ability to control the response.

2.5. Discrimination Training

Another innovation in the study of interoceptive stimuli has been to train discrimination. This is important for two reasons. First, it permits one to estimate the physiological limits of discrimination. Differences between people in their awareness of a gastrointestinal stimulus may represent differences in their learning history or physical differences between them. Discrimination training provides a way of separating these two influences. Stunkard and Fox (1971) taught human subjects to discriminate stomach contractions which they could not previously discriminate, and Ádám (1967) taught a human subject to discriminate the occurrence of balloon distension of the jejunum at volumes which previously had elicited alpha EEG blocking but no reliable verbal reports.

The second advantage of training discrimination is that it permits one to use animals to study visceral perception. Slucki, Ádám, and Porter (1965) demonstrated that rhythmic inflation of a balloon in an isolated loop of small intestine could be made the discriminative stimulus controlling lever-pressing behavior in the rhesus monkey. They later repeated this using an isolated loop of descending colon as the site of stimulation (Slucki, McCoy, & Porter, 1969). The importance of being able to use animals in the study of visceral perception is that they can be studied over an extended period of time, and the pathways subserving visceral perception can be studied by sectioning.

3. Behavioral Significance of Visceral Perception

In the introduction to this chapter, it was pointed out (1) that people are aware of some events occurring in the gastrointestinal tract, (2) that the types of events which are perceived represent a selected subset of afferent information available to the brain from the gut, (3) that there are individual differences in ability to perceive gastrointestinal stimuli, and (4) that the discriminability of these stimuli improves with training. This combination of circumstances is probably meaningful rather than coincidental, and it suggests that visceral perception plays a role in the organism's behavioral adjustment to its environment. Several hypotheses about what that role is have been advanced, and these hypotheses are reviewed in the next sections.

3.1. Cuing Function in Bowel Control

The most thoroughly investigated and best documented hypothesis is that the perception of rectal distension serves as a cue to the organism to emit certain behaviors which result in (1) the temporary withholding of a bowel movement and (2) the seeking out of an appropriate place in which to defecate. The temporary withholding or postponement of a bowel movement is achieved by a phasic contraction of the external anal sphincter during the period in which the internal anal sphincter is reflexly inhibited by rectal distension. Although this phasic contraction has occasionally been referred to as a reflex (Alva, Mendeloff, & Schuster, 1967), the bulk of evidence suggests that it is a voluntary response (Whitehead, Orr, Engel, & Schuster, 1981). For example, Rodriquez and Awad (1979) have reported that the phasic external anal sphincter contraction does not occur in response to rectal distension in spinal cord transected patients even though reflex inhibition of the internal anal sphincter in response to rectal distension does occur in such patients. Melzak and Porter (1964) reported some years ago that rectal distension did produce external sphincter contraction in spinal cord transected patients. However, their records show very brief electrical potentials which could have been artifactually produced by movement of the tissue relative to their rigid needle electrodes.

Loss of sensation in the rectum as a result of surgery or injury is frequently associated with incontinence of stool (Cerulli, Nikoomanesh, & Schuster, 1979; Goligher & Hughes, 1951). Moreover, in our biofeedback clinic for the treatment of fecal incontinence, we find that patients who are not able to perceive at least 15 ml of air injected into a balloon never achieved continence, whereas most of the patients who can perceive smaller amounts of rectal distension do benefit from biofeedback training (Whitehead, Engel, & Schuster, 1981). The normal threshold of rectal distension which is perceived is 5 ml in our laboratory.

3.2. Hunger and Satiety

Both Hertz (1911) and Cannon and Washburn (1912) stated that contractions of the stomach give rise to sensations of hunger. Hertz based his conclusions on anecdotal evidence, but Cannon and Washburn recorded contractions by means of a large balloon in the stomach and observed that subjects were more likely to report hunger during periods of gastric motility than during its absence.

Stunkard and his co-workers (Griggs & Stunkard, 1964; Stunkard & Koch, 1964; Stunkard & Fox, 1971) were the first to investigate this hypothesis systematically. Their initial studies appeared to confirm the association between hunger and gastric motility in normal subjects, and they generated much excitement by their data which showed that obese subjects gave reports of hunger which were uncorrelated with gastric motility. This suggested that either inability to discriminate gastric contractions or inappropriate labeling of gastric contractions might explain obesity.

Unfortunately, Stunkard's subsequent experiments (Stunkard & Fox, 1971) did not confirm these early impressions. Stunkard found that when subjects were asked to rate the intensity of their hunger rather than to respond "yes" or "no" and when subjects were run for longer period of observation, the association between hunger and gastric motility was weak and inconstant. Only 25% of subjects showed a strong association between hunger ratings and gastric motility, and this association was variable from one occasion of testing to another. Moreover, training subjects to be more accurate discriminators of gastric contractions did not improve the strength of the association between gastric contractions and hunger ratings and did not enable obese subjects to regulate food intake more effectively.

These observations are consistent with the effects of vagotomy (Grossman, Cummins, & Ivy, 1947), which eliminates sensations from the stomach, and gastrectomy (MacDonald, Inglefinger, & Belding, 1947), which eliminates gastric motility. Subjects continue to experience hunger after both types of surgery. Stunkard and Fox (1971) concluded that there is, in fact, an association between subjectively more potent determinants of hunger. They suggest that earlier studies overestimated the strength of this relationship between hunger and motility because they used insensitive measures of hunger; there is a strong tendency for hunger to increase over time from the end of one meal to the beginning of the next, and this tendency may reduce the probability of discovering a lack of association between the two variables.

Whitehead and Drescher (1980) assessed awareness of stomach contractions in 20 normal subjects and asked them to describe all the cues they used to determine when their stomach was contracting. The most common cues mentioned were a tight feeling in the stomach (16/20) and stomach noises (15/20). Only 3 subjects in 20 mentioned hunger sensations, and none of these felt that "hunger pangs" were the most helpful cue for solving the discrimination task.

Sensations arising in the stomach have also been implicated in satiety and the cessation of eating. Hertz (1911) stated that distension of the stomach produced a feeling of fullness which led to the cessation of eating. Deutsch, Young, and Kalogeris (1978) confirmed in an elegant series of experiments that distension of the stomach does play a critical role in regulating the volume of food eaten. They implanted an inflatable cuff around the pylorus of rats to enable them to separate gastric from duodenal stimulation, and they implanted a gastric canula. They were able to show that rats eat a fixed volume of a familiar liquid diet and that withdrawal of part of the stomach contents after the rat has eaten to satiety will cause him to resume eating and to eat enough to replace the amount removed. This quantitative relationship between gastric filling volume and eating behaviors was observed whether or not food was allowed to enter the duodenum.

McHugh (1979) has shown that under normal circumstances gastric distension is a function of gastric emptying rate, and that gastric emptying is a regulated process, the speed of which is determined by the caloric content of the meal. The first part of a meal enters the duodenum where the caloric content of the meal is sensed, and gastric emptying is inhibited proportional to caloric concentration.

This experimental work on the role of gastric distension in eating behavior is supported by clinical observations on gastrectomized patients (MacDonald, Inglefinger, & Belding, 1947). These individuals, in whom stomach distension does not occur or cannot be signaled to the brain, tend to overeat.

Although these observations demonstrate that afferent information from the stomach controls cessation of eating, they do not indicate how this occurs. Hertz (1911) implied that one feels the distension of his stomach directly as fullness and labels it as repletion. However, Garcia, Hankins, and Rusiniak (1974) have suggested that gastric distension controls eating indirectly by modifying the hedonic value of food, that is, whether the taste is preferred. The experimental literature on the reinforcing value of intragastric feeding and on conditioned taste aversions and conditioned taste preferences (see p. 341) supports Garcia's hedonic shift hypothesis.

Several experiments have addressed the question of whether food injected directly into the stomachs of rats will serve as a reinforcer which maintains lever-pressing behavior because this experiment appears to differentiate between drive reduction and hedonic theories of reinforcement. Most of these studies found that intragastric reinforcement would maintain behavior on which it was contingent. However, Holman (1968) demonstrated that intragastric feeding would reinforce lever-pressing behavior only if there was concurrent stimulation of some type to the palate or throat. This oral stimulation could be nothing more than a change in the palate or throat. This oral stimulation could be nothing more than a change in temperature. Holman showed that rats previously trained to press a bar for food would extinguish if they were provided with contingent oral stimulation but no intragastric nutrient, and they would extinguish if provided with contingent intragastric feeding but no oral stimulation. Both cues presented together, however, would maintain the lever-pressing behavior. This outcome is consistent with Garcia's hypothesis that gastrointestinal stimuli exert an influence on behavior which is not mediated by their direct perception but rather is mediated by hedonic shift in gustatory or related oral stimuli.

Similar conclusions can be drawn from the conditioned taste aversion literature. The general finding is that illness produced by radiation or by lithium chloride ingestion causes the animal to develop conditioned taste aversions to any novel taste which has preceded the illness. Similarly, the animal will develop conditioned taste preferences for any taste which precedes the recovery from illness or recovery from vitamin deficiency. There are several interesting aspects to such conditioning, including the fact that learning occurs even when long delays occur between the gustatory stimulus and the illness, and the fact that the aversion is developed specifically to the taste cue rather than to the place where the food was eaten or to its physical appearance.

Many of the illness-producing agents which Garcia used (e.g., radiation) are not specific to the gastrointestinal tract; he refers to interoceptive stimuli generally as exerting their effects on behavior through shifts in incentive, motivation, or hedonic value.

It is important to note that Garcia's hypothesis does not require that the subject be aware of the interoceptive stimulus or even that he be aware of the hedonic shift in taste for the conditioned taste aversion to develop. Garcia has shown that conditioned taste aversions develop when illness occurs during unconsciousness produced by anesthesia or by chemically-induced cortical depression. This suggests that perception plays little or no role in the effects on eating behavior of afferent information from the gut. Whether actual perception would add anything to the precision of behavioral self-regulation of the internal environment remains to be investigated.

3.3. Labeling of Emotions

The most popular view of the significance of visceral perception is that these sensations represent self-perceptions of emotional arousal. This theory was first formalized by William James (1884) and Lange (1922), and despite empirical data which tended to discredit the theory (Cannon, 1927), the so-called James-Lange theory of emotion continues to attract adherents. It strongly influenced psychoanalytic thinking about psychosomatic etiology. For example, the 1968 edition of the *Diagnostic and Statistical Manual of Mental Disorders* held that psychosomatic symptoms were the normal physiological manifestations of chronic emotional states. The emotions which were said to be associated with gastrointestinal activity included dependency and an angry desire to get revenge in the case of peptic ulcer and hopelessness or humiliation in the case of ulcerative colitis (Alexander, French, & Pollock, 1968; Graham, Lundy, Benjamin, Kabler, Lewis, Kunish, & Graham, 1962).

A modified version of the James-Lange theory of emotion was proposed by Schachter and Singer (1962) and dubbed attribution theory. They argued that awareness of his own autonomic arousal leads the subject to conclude that he is experiencing an emotion, but the subject depends on cognitive cues from the environment such as the behavior of other people or past experience to determine the type of emotion which is occurring.

Attribution theory seems to agree well with most of the available experimental literature. The Schachter and Singer (1962) experiments, which manipulated autonomic arousal by injecting epinephrine and also manipulated cognitive cues, indicated that the injection of epinephrine contributed to the perceived intensity but not to the identity of the emotions which subjects reported. Hohmann's (1966) observations on changes in the emotional experiences of spinal cord transected patients indicated that there is a decrease in the perceived intensity of emotional reactions after injury. The magnitude of the decrease is proportional to the level of the lesion and, therefore, to the amount of decrease in autonomic arousal and sensory feedback about autonomic arousal.

There are few data in the literature which bear directly on the emotional significance which subjects attach to perceptions of gastrointestinal responses. Ádám (1974) has done experiments in animals which suggest that mild stimulation of the gastrointestinal tract dampens negative emotional states and/or induces sleep whereas strong stimulation of the gastrointestinal tract may be perceived as aversive. In our experiments investigating the ability of human subjects to detect spontaneous contractions of their stomachs or distension of a small balloon in their colon, subjects have never described these stimuli in affective terms. Stomach contractions are typically described as a tensing or squeezing sensation in the abdomen, and distension of the colon is described as a feeling like gas distension. However, the experimental setting may have mitigated against subjects' interpreting their perceptions as emotional arousal.

Some incidental observations in our study of stomach contractions are relevant to the hypothesis that perceptions of autonomic responses may contribute to the self-attribution of emotion. We observed a small but statistically significant correlation ($r = .51$) between subjects' ability to perceive stomach contractions and their ability to perceive heart beats. This suggests a generalized tendency to be aware of, or to attend to, internal events, which would appear to be one of the requirements of any theory of emotion which treats self-perceptions as an important determinant. We also observed that men are significantly better than women, on average, at discriminating both stomach contractions and heart beats. The significance of this is unknown.

To summarize the discussion of emotional labeling, it appears that perception of gastrointestinal activity may lead people to attribute emotions to themselves, but this has not been directly verified. It is clear that people do not invariably attribute emotional arousal to their perceptions of gastrointestinal activity; they are capable of attributing these sensations to something they ate, something the investigator did to them, or to disease.

3.4. Acquisition and Retention of Voluntary Control over a Visceral Response

Brener (1974a,b; 1977a,b) proposed a specific role for visceral perception in the acquisition of self-control over a visceral response. He theorized that in order to emit any voluntary act the brain calls up an image of the sensory consequences associated with the response and then executes motor acts until the sensory feedback from the target organ (such as the heart) corresponds to the stored image of what those sensations should be. This theory is derived from William James's (1890) ideomotor theory of voluntary acts. From this, Brener inferred that learning to discriminate the sensory consequences associated with a visceral response is both necessary and sufficient to enable the subject to emit the response on command as a voluntary response. Biofeedback training, according to Brener, is discrimination training in which the subject learns to correctly identify and label the sensations associated with the response he is attempting to learn how to produce.

Brener's theory has a number of practical implications. Not only does it appear to explain biofeedback learning, but it also suggests ways in which biofeedback training might be made more effective. It suggests, for example, that eliciting large-magnitude changes in the visceral response by means of unconditional stimuli while providing feedback would be more effective than the usual procedure of advising the subject to sit quietly and concentrate on the feedback.

Several investigators have reported experimental tests of Brener's theory. Most of these have compared heart beat perception to heart rate control. Some studies have supported the theory (Clemens, 1976; Clemens & MacDonald, 1976; McFarland, 1975), while others have not (Dale & Anderson, 1978; Whitehead, Drescher, Heiman, & Blackwell, 1977).

Whitehead and Drescher (1980) suggested that the inconsistent outcomes in tests of Brener's theory have resulted because heart rate is a poor choice of systems in which to test the theory. We noted that within the normal range of values heart rate is closely linked to respiration, and that this permitted subjects in some experiments to solve the perception task by manipulating their breathing (Ross & Brener, 1981). In other experiments the perception task was insensitive to respiration-induced heart rate changes. A second problem with heart rate is that subjects already know a variety of strategies include changing respiration, tensing muscles, and using cognitive imagery of stimuli or events which unconditionally elicit heart rate changes. Some of the methods of heart rate control may by related to heart rate perception while other are not. Whitehead and Drescher (1980) suggested that this difficulty can be solved by switching to a new response system, gastric motility, which is not elicited by any known skeletal muscle response and which subjects initially have little ability to control.

In the experiment reported by Whitehead and Drescher (1980) subjects were tested for ability to detect individual contractions of their stomachs. Contractions were recorded as changes in intragastric pressure measured with a perfused catheter. On each of approximately 200 trials, which occurred over six 2-hr sessions, the experimenter turned on a light either at the peak of a stomach contraction or approximately 12 sec following the peak of a contraction. The subject had to indicate on each trial whether he thought the signal light coincided with a stomach contraction. The subject's responses were analyzed by the method of signal detection.

Following the perception test, subjects were asked to increase and decrease their stomach motility prior to feedback training. Then, half the subjects were given biofeedback training to control motility while the other half practiced without feedback. The feedback subjects acquired the ability to increase motility during feedback training but could not reduce motility below resting levels. The no-feedback subjects did not acquire control over gastric motility. With respect to Brener's theory, the control of gastric motility was not correlated with individual differences in the ability to perceive gastric contractions either before biofeedback training or at the end of feedback training. This occurred even though half the subjects could perceive stomach contractions at better than chance levels.

Brener's theory of voluntary visceral control is not supported by these data. However, Brener (Ross & Brener, 1981) has recently revised the theory to state that the sensory information which is critical to self-control of a visceral response is not peripheral receptor activity but central efferent monitoring of the brain's motor commands to the viscera. This new formulation of the theory has not been tested experimentally.

In addition to Brener's theory of visceral response acquisition, Weiss and Engel (1971) have proposed that accurate perception of a visceral response learned during biofeedback training may be critical to retention of the response. The reasoning is that if the subject can perceive when he has successfully emitted the response there is secondary reinforcement for the performance, but if the subject cannot perceive the occurrence of the response there will be no reinforcement and the response will extinguish. This plausible hypothesis has not been tested.

3.5. Psychosomatic Etiology

A hypothesis similar to Brener's was advanced by White-head, Fedoravicius, Blackwell, and Wooley (1979) to account for the etiology of some types of psychosomatic disorders. This hypothesis owed much to Miller (1977), who had argued that pathophysiological responses underlying many psychosomatic disorders might be inadvertently learned through social reinforcement in the same way that biofeedback training explicitly teaches the subject to modify a physiological response by providing contingent information or rewards. The analogy which Miller used was that a child who is given special attention and allowed to stay home from school when he has a stomachache but not when he has a headache may learn to emit at a greater frequency and a greater amplitude the pathophysiological responses (such as gastric acid secretion) which produced the stomachache. Such a child, Miller proposed, might grow up to have an ulcer.

Whitehead et al. (1979) pointed out that this sequence of events could only occur if the subject perceived the pathophysiological response and reported it accurately. Other people in the environment can only reinforce verbal behavior or overt physiological events. If the subject is unaware of when a physiological event is occurring or if he complains at times when it is not occurring, the social reinforcement which he receives contingent on somatic complaints might increase the frequency of complaints but could not reinforce physiological changes. On the other hand, accurate reports of physiological changes could be rewarded in such a way that the reinforcer is temporally close to the physiological change and reinforces it.

This hypothesis led Whitehead et al. to make two predictions: (1) Individuals with certain psychosomatic disorders would show greater awareness of the associated physiological response than would individuals without the disorder, and (2) psychosomatic disorders associated with easily perceived pathophysiological responses would be more likely to exhibit a history of control by social reinforcement than would difficult-to-perceive responses.

The first prediction appeared to be supported by Ritchie's (1973) data on irritable bowel syndrome. He found that when he distended the colon with a balloon, patients with irritable bowel syndrome reported pain at a lower threshold of distension than did normal controls. We attempted to replicate this finding and to evaluate the threshold for perceiving any distension in patients with irritable bowel syndrome and in normals (Whitehead, Engel, & Schuster, 1980). We did replicate Ritchie's finding that patients were significantly more likely to report pain with moderate amounts of distension than were normal subjects. However, we were not able to test the hypothesis that the patients could detect weaker stimuli than the normal subjects because we could not find a weak enough stimulus to measure any individual differences. Our apparatus consisted of a flaccid balloon 5 cm long which was placed in the rectosigmoid junction. The smallest amount of air which we could reliably inject into this balloon to stimulate the bowel was 5 ml. Nearly all the patients and normal subjects could detect this weak stimulus on 100% of trials. While we could conceivably have made the discrimination test more sensitive by using 2-point discrimination or by inflating the balloon more slowly, we reasoned that any differences between patients and normal which might be discovered in this way were too small to be of physiological or psychological significance. Most subjects appear capable of feeling just about every contraction of their bowel if they attend to it.

We have also found that perceptual sensitivity is excellent in the small intestine. In two patients with ileostomies, we inserted small balloons 5–10 cm into the stoma and found that they could invariably detect the addition of 2.5 ml of air to these balloons.

The second prediction referred to previously was that disorders associated with easily perceived pathophysiological responses should show more evidence of control by social reinforcement than disorders associated with difficult to perceive physiological responses. This question was investigated in an epidemiological survey (Whitehead, Winget, Fedoravicius, Wooley, & Blackwell, 1982) in which we compared patients with irritable bowel syndrome to those with peptic ulcer. Gastric acid secretion, which is the presumed pathophysiological response for peptic ulcer, is very difficult to perceive.

In the epidemiological survey we asked people what illnesses they had and how they treated themselves, and we also asked them whether their parents had rewarded them when they were ill as children. Significantly larger proportions of patients with irritable bowel syndrome as compared to peptic ulcer exhibited chronic illness behavior. They were more likely to report multiple somatic complaints, they believed their colds were more frequent and more serious than those of other people, and they were more likely to go to a doctor for treatment of a cold rather than to treat it themselves. These chronic illness behaviors were shown to be linked to the childhood reinforcement of illness in the form of gifts and special consideration. Patients with irritable bowel syndrome were significantly more likely than people without this disorder to report that their parents rewarded them for illness. This was not true of people with peptic ulcer. These data tend to confirm the prediction that an easily perceived pathophysiological response is more likely to come under the control of social reinforcers than a difficult-to-perceive response.

4. Summary and Conclusions

This review of the behavioral significance of sensations arising in the gastrointestinal tract suggests that these sensations fulfill two very different functional roles. They may serve as discriminative stimuli which are directly perceived and which signal the occasion for behavioral interactions with the social environment. Alternatively, sensory information from the gut may act indirectly on behavior by modifying the incentive value of foods so as to maintain a constant internal envrionment.

Perhaps the best example of the discriminative stimulus function of gastrointestinal stimuli is the urge to defecate which is produced by rectal distension and which enables the individual to postpone defecation until he can find a socially appropriate place. Another instance of this discriminative stimulus function is when self-perceptions of autonomic arousal lead people to infer that they are emotionally aroused but do not determine what emotion they are feeling; they must apparently depend on prior experience, expectations, and the behavior of others to decide whether they are actually emotionally aroused or just sick and what the emotion is that they are experiencing. The hypothesized role of awareness in psychosomatic etiology can also be grouped under discriminative stimulus functions: The perception of a certain gastrointestinal response is the stimulus in the presence of which a verbal complaint may be reinforced.

It is apparently the case that gastrointestinal sensations which serve as discriminative stimuli must be actually perceived in order for the subject to respond to them. This distinguishes them from the second type of sensation referred to above which may exert its influence on behavior even if the subject is unconscious during the time the stimulus (e.g., illness) occurs. A second distinction is that discriminative stimuli cue behaviors which involve interactions with the external environment but have nothing directly to do with the internal environment. The second category of sensory events, on the other hand, are exclusively concerned with the internal environment.

Perceptual sensitivity for the gastrointestinal sensations which serve as discriminative stimuli can be improved with discrimination training. It is interesting to speculate on just how much awareness of the events in one's gastrointestinal tract could be achieved with such training. There may be additional unsuspected opportunities for these sensations to serve as discriminative stimuli.

The other kind of functional role which gastrointestinal stimuli can serve, namely, the modification of the incentive properties of food, is exemplified by the role of gastric distension in satiety. Garcia argues that satiety and the cessation of eating is mediated exclusively by hedonic shifts in the taste of foods. Other examples are the reinforcing value of food, which seems to depend on a combination of oral stimulation and gastrointestinal stimulation; and the development of conditioned taste aversions and taste preferences.

It appears that perception of gastrointestinal responses is not essential to learning to voluntarily control these responses during biofeedback training. Garcia et al. (1974) even suggest that visceral sensations cannot be utilized in the learning of instrumental responses, and indeed biofeedback training of visceral responses almost invariably involves the use of visual or auditory feedback signals to indicate what is happening to a visceral process. Garcia may be right that only such exteroceptive channels of information can be used to establish instrumental responses. This remains to be determined.

A relatively large number of gastrointestinal sensations which we know are discriminable are left with no assigned role by this review and summary. Examples are the sensitivity of the esophagus to temperature and the sensitivity of the stomach and intestines to distension. Since evolutionary selection is rarely so promiscuous as to give an organism sensory modalities which are unrelated to survival, it is likely that gastrointestinal sensations serve important functions in behavioral regulation which are as yet not understood.

The gastrointestinal tract seems to be more richly endowed with sensations that reach awareness than other visceral systems, for example, the cardiovascular system. Perhaps this is because the gastrointestinal tract is actually a body surface like the skin which is in contact with a variable environment. The body may need extrasensory and response capabilities to be able to deal flexibly with the unpredictable environment found in the gut so as to avoid or rapidly eliminate toxins and parasites while maintaining an adequate supply of nutrition.

References

Ádám, G. (1967). *Interoception and behavior*. Budapest: Akadémiai Kiadó.

Ádám, G. (1974). Interoceptive stimuli and learning. In *Proceedings of the International Union of Physiological Sciences* (Vol. 10). New Delhi: Core Book Programme of the Government of India.

Alexander, F., French, T. M., & Pollock, G. (1968). *Psychosomatic specificity: Experimental study and results* (Vol. 1). Chicago: University of Chicago Press.

Alva, J., Mendeloff, A. I., & Schuster, M. M. (1967). Reflex and electromyographic abnormalities associated with fecal incontinence. *Gastroenterology, 53*, 101–106.

American Psychiatric Association (1968). *Diagnostic and statistical manual of mental disorders* (2nd ed.). Washington, DC: APA.

Brener, J. (1974a). A general model of voluntary control applied to the phenomena of learned cardiovascular change. In P. A. Obrist, A. H. Black, J. Brener, & L. V. DiCara (Eds.), *Cardiovascular psychophysiology*. Chicago: Aldine.

Brener, J. (1974b). Factors influencing the specificity of voluntary cardiovascular control. In L. V. DiCara (Ed.), *Limbic and autonomic nervous systems research*. New York: Plenum Press.

Brener, J. (1977a). Sensory and perceptual determinants of voluntary visceral control. In G. E. Schwartz & J. Beatty (Eds.), *Biofeedback: Theory and research.* New York: Academic Press.

Brener, J. (1977b). Visceral perception. In J. Beatty & H. Legwie (Eds.), *Biofeedback and behavior.* New York: Plenum Press.

Brener, J., & Jones, J. M. (1974). Interoceptive discrimination in intact humans: Detection of cardiac activity. *Physiology and Behavior, 13,* 763–767.

Bruner, J. S., & Postman, L. (1947). Emotional selectivity in perception and reaction. *Journal of Personality, 16,* 69–77.

Cannon, W. B. (1927). The James-Lange theory of emotion. *American Journal of Psychology, 39,* 106–124.

Cannon, W. B., & Washburn, A. A. (1912). An explanation of hunger. *American Journal of Physiology, 29,* 441–454.

Cerulli, M. A., Nikoomanesh, P., & Schuster, M. M. (1979). Progress in biofeedback conditioning for fecal incontinence. *Gastroenterology, 76,* 742–746.

Clemens, W. J. (1976). *Heart beat discrimination and the learning and transfer of voluntary heart rate control.* Paper presented at the Southeastern Psychological Association meeting, New Orleans, March.

Clemens, W. J., & MacDonald, D. F. (1976). Relationship between heart beat discrimination and heart rate control. *Psychophysiology, 13,* 176.

Dale, A., & Anderson, D. (1978). Information variables in voluntary control and classical conditioning of heart rate: Field dependence and heart-rate perception. *Perceptual and Motor Skills, 47,* 79–85.

Deutsch, J. A., Young, W. G., & Kalogeris, T. J. (1978). The stomach signals satiety. *Science, 201,* 165–167.

Garcia, J., Hankins, W. G., & Rusiniak, K. W. (1974). Behavioral regulation of the milieu interne in man and rat. *Science, 185,* 824–831.

Goligher, J. C., & Hughes, E. S. R. (1951). Sensibility of the rectum and colon: Its role in the mechanism of anal continence. *Lancet, 1,* 543–548.

Graham, D. T., Lundy, R. M., Benjamin, L. S., Kabler, J. D., Lewis, W. C., Kunish, N. D., & Graham, F. K. (1962). Specific attitudes in initial interviews with patients having different "psychosomatic diseases." *Psychosomatic Medicine, 24,* 257–266.

Griggs, R. C., & Stunkard, A. (1964). The interpretation of gastric motility. II. Sensitivity and bias in the perception of gastric motility. *Archives of General Psychiatry, 11,* 82–89.

Grossman, M. I., Cummins, G. M., & Ivy, A. C. (1947). The effect of insulin on food intake after vagotomy and sympathectomy. *American Journal of Physiology, 149,* 100–102.

Hefferline, A. F., Keenan, B., & Harford, R. A. (1956). Escape and avoidance conditioning in human subjects without their observation of the response. *Science, 130,* 1338–1339.

Hertz, A. F. (1911). *The sensibility of the alimentary canal.* London: Oxford University Press.

Hohmann, G. W. (1966). Some effects of spinal cord lesions on experienced emotional feelings. *Psychophysiology, 3*, 143–156.

Holman, G. L. (1968). Intragastric reinforcement effect. *Journal of Comparative and Physiological Psychology, 69*, 432–441.

Iggo, A. (1957). Gastric mucosal chemoreceptors with vagal afferent fibers in the cat. *Quarterly Journal of Experimental Physiology, 42*, 398–409.

James, W. (1890). *The principles of psychology*. New York: Henry Holt.

James, W. (1884). What is emotion? *Mind, 19*, 188–205.

Lange, C. (1922). The emotions (I. A. Haupt., Trans.). In K. Dunlap (Ed.), *The emotions*. Baltimore: Williams & Wilkins.

Leek, B. F. (1972). Abdominal visceral receptors. In E. Neil (Ed.), *Enteroceptors: Handbook of sensory physiology* (Vol. 3, No. 1). New York: Springer-Verlag.

MacDonald, R. M., Inglefinger, F. J., & Belding, H. Z. W. (1947). Late effects of total gastrectomy in man. *New England Journal of Medicine, 237*, 887–896.

McFarland, R. A. (1975). Heart rate perception and heart rate control. *Psychophysiology, 12*, 402–405.

McHugh, P. R. (1979). Aspects of the control of feeding: Application of quantitation in psychobiology. *Johns Hopkins Medical Journal, 144*, 147–155.

Melzak, I., & Porter, N. H. (1964). Studies of the reflex activity of the external sphincter ani in spinal man. *Paraplegia, 1*, 277–296.

Miller, N. E. (1977). Effect of learning on gastrointestinal functions. *Clinics in Gastroenterology, 6*, 533–546.

Ritchie, J. (1973). Pain from distension of the pelvic colon by inflating a balloon in the irritable colon syndrome. *Gut, 14*, 125–132.

Rodriquez, A. A., & Awad, E. (1979). Detrusor muscle and sphincteric response to anorectal stimulation in spinal cord injury. *Archives of Physical Medicine and Rehabilitation, 60*, 269–272.

Ross, A., & Brener, J. (1981). Two procedures for training cardiac discrimination. A comparison of solution strategies and their relationship to heart rate control. *Psychophysiology, 18*, 62–70.

Schachter, A., & Singer, J. E. (1962). Cognitive, social, and psychological determinants of emotional state. *Psychological Review, 69*, 379–399.

Slucki, H., Ádám, G., & Porter, R. W. (1965). Operant discrimination of an interoceptive stimulus in rhesus monkeys. *Journal of the Experimental Analysis of Behavior, 8*, 405–414.

Slucki, H., McCoy, F. B., & Porter, R. W. (1969). Interoceptive S^D of the large intestine established by mechanical stimulation. *Psychological Reports, 24*, 35–42.

Stunkard, A. J., & Fox, S. (1971). The relationship of gastric motility and hunger: A summary of the evidence. *Psychosomatic Medicine, 33*, 123–134.

Stunkard, A. J., & Koch, C. (1964). The interpretation of gastric motility. I. Apparent bias in the reports of hunger by obese persons. *Archives of General Psychiatry, 11*, 74–82.

Swets, J. A. (1973). The relative operating characteristic in psychology. *Science, 182*, 990–1000.

Tanner, W. E., & Swets, J. A. (1954). A decision-making theory of visual detection. *Psychological Review, 61*, 401–409.

Weiss, T., & Engel, B. T. (1971). Operant conditioning of heart rate in patients with premature ventricular contractions. *Psychosomatic Medicine, 33*, 301–321.

Whitehead, W. E., & Drescher, V. M. (1980). Perception of gastric contractions and self-control of gastric motility. *Psychophysiology, 17*, 552–558.

Whitehead, W. E., Drescher, V. M., Heiman, P., & Blackwell, B. (1977). Relation of heart rate control to heart beat perception. *Biofeedback and Self-Regulation, 2*, 371–392.

Whitehead, W. E., Engel, B. T., & Schuster, M. M. (1980). Irritable bowel syndrome: Physiological and psychological differences between diarrhea-predominant and constipation-predominant patients. *Digestive Diseases and Sciences, 25*, 404–413.

Whitehead, W. E., Engel, B. T., & Schuster, M. M. (1981). Perception of rectal distension is necessary to prevent fecal incontinence. In G. Ádám, I. Meszaros, & E. I. Banyai (Eds.), *Advances in physiological sciences* (Vol. 17). *Brain and Behavior.* Budapest, Hungary: Akadémiai Kiadó.

Whitehead, W. E., Fedoravicius, A. S., Blackwell, B., & Wooley, S. (1979). Psychosomatic symptoms as learned responses. In J. R. McNamara (Ed.), *Behavioral approaches in medicine: Application and analysis.* New York: Plenum Press.

Whitehead, W. E., Orr, W. C., Engel, B. T., & Schuster, M. M. (1981). External anal sphincter response to rectal distension: Learned response or reflex. *Psychophysiology, 19*, 57–62.

Whitehead, W. E., Winget, C., Fedoravicius, A. S., Wooley, S., & Blackwell, B. (1982). Learned illness behavior in patients with irritable bowel syndrome and peptic ulcer. *Digestive Diseases and Sciences, 27*, 202–208.

APPENDIX *III*

Learning to Perceive Previously Unconscious Stimuli

A simple form of the unconscious is when a person cannot perceive a stimulus. The stimulus is physically there but the person has not learned to discriminate or perceive it. In a tropical rain forest, a guide points to where a bird is in a tangle of trees. The novice's eyes are stimulated by the same pattern of light as the guide's, but he does not see any bird. With enough training, he becomes better able to perceive birds in the forest. In a Ph.D. dissertation with me, Douglas Lawrence (1948) showed that it is much easier to teach subjects to perceive a small difference if one starts out with a large one first and progressively proceeds to smaller ones than if one gives the same number of trials all on the difficult discrimination. The nature guide does something like this when he focuses his spotting telescope on the bird for the novice to look through. More systematic training using a zoom lens might be even more helpful.

From Neal E. Miller: Some examples of psychophysiology and the unconscious. *Biofeedback and Self-Regulation, 17,* 3–16, 1992.

Inhibition of Alpha Waves: An Index of Ability to Learn a Perception

Ordinarily many visceral conditions are poorly perceived, but with a number of them, patients can be trained to discriminate so that they become conscious of them. In Hungary Professor George Ádám (1967) trained animals and people to respond correctly to various types of visceral stimulation. In one experiment he had human subjects swallow a thin tube ending in a small balloon. It was inserted until x-rays showed that the balloon was in the duodenal region of the intestine. Then he had each subject relax until a consistent series of high-voltage, low-frequency alpha waves appeared in the EEG recordings from electrodes on the skull. These waves indicate a low level of arousal. But as soon as a new stimulus is presented, arousal of the reticular formation inhibits these brain waves and replaces them with low-voltage high-frequency ones. He used this phenomenon to determine the threshold for the amount of inflation of the balloon that would activate the reticular formation as indicated by inhibition of the alpha waves. At this level the subject could not discriminate (i.e., verbally report) the inflation of the balloon. Then the amount of inflation was increased in 5–10 mm Hg steps until the subject reached the initial threshold of detecting the stimulation.

After this the balloon was deflated, and when the alpha waves reappeared the procedure was repeated for a number of what Ádám describes as verbally reinforced conditioning trials in which the subject was told: "The intestinal stimulus is now applied." Such training progressively reduced the threshold for perceiving the distention, which remained low, often at a level approximating the threshold for inhibiting alpha waves, even after the experimenter's verbal reinforcements were discontinued. It is significant that initially the response of a lower level of the brain, the reticular formation responsible for inhibiting alpha waves to a novel stimulus, occurred even when the subject was unable to report perceiving the stimulus and that with practice the subjects became better able to perceive the visceral stimulus.

These and other experiments by Ádám indicate that the inhibition of alpha waves may be useful for basic research and for diagnosing whether or not a patient is likely to be able to learn therapeutic perception of a specific visceral stimulus.

Unconscious Learning

Can there be unconscious learning? According to an early version of cognitive theory, all learned behavior results from acquiring knowledge of what leads to what (Tolman, 1932). Then consciousness of this correct knowledge leads to the performance of the correct response. From this point of view, there could be no unconscious learning or even completely unconscious performance. This view led to a considerable controversy over whether learning could occur without awareness. Strong evidence against such an extreme cognitive view comes from the case of H. M., a patient with bilateral lesions in the hippocampus and the amygdala who suffered from extreme memory defects. Given trials on a mirror drawing task on a number of different days, at each session he convincingly demonstrated failure to show any glimmer of recognition of ever having seen the room, the task, or the experimenter. But, over a series of sessions he showed definite improvement. This demonstrated unconscious results of learning. In other types of situations he failed to show any learning; the difference between the tasks that he could and could not learn merits discussion beyond the scope of this article (Milner, 1962; Cohen and Squire, 1980).

To give another example, once I suffered a strain of the muscles in my right arm and shoulder which made certain movements quite painful without eliminating the possibility of making them. Later, when I had occasion to see a doctor about a few lingering pains, he asked me to raise my hands above my head. I was utterly astonished that I could not raise my right arm above the horizontal. The pain had motivated—and escape from pain reinforced—learning not to try to reach up with my right hand and instead to reach up with my left, but I was not at all conscious of such learning. Absence of reaching up during recovery from injury caused adhesions to form that produced the deficit. Fortunately, suitable exercise corrected it. During the early part of this unconscious learning and performance, it was adaptive in saving me from pain; as conditions changed it became maladaptive in allowing the adhesions to form.

Many completely irrational emotional responses such as strong fear of mice or great uneasiness in the presence of heights, even though a glass window may safely separate one from the abyss below, are elicited without a conscious reason. The situation is encapsulated in the quotation: "I do not like thee Dr. Fell, the reason why I cannot tell, but this I know and know full well, I do not like thee Dr. Fell."

References

Ádám, G. (1967). Interoception and behaviour. Budapest: Akadémiai Kiadó.

Cohen, N. J., & Squire, L. R. (1980). Preserved learning and retention of pattern-analyzing skill in amnesia: Dissociation of knowing how and knowing that. Science, 210, 207–209.

Lawrence, D. H. (1948). The acquired distinctiveness of cues. Partially unpublished Yale University dissertation.

Milner, B. (1962). Les troubles de la memoire accompagnant des lesions hippocampques bilaterales. In Physiologie de l'hippocampe (pp. 257–272). Paris: CNRS.

Tolman, E.C. (1932). Purposive behavior in animals and men. New York and London: The Century Co.

References

Ábrahám, A. (1949). Receptors in the wall of the blood vessels. *Acta Biol. Acad. Sci. Hung. 1*, 157.

Ábrahám, A. (1964). *Die mikroskopische Innervation des Herzens und der Blutgefässe von Vertebraten*. Budapest: Akadémiai Kiadó.

Accarino, A. M., Azpiroz, F., & Malagelada, J. R. (1995). Selective dysfunction of mechanosensitive intestinal afferents in irritable bowel syndrome. *Gastroenterology, 108,* 636–643.

Acker, H. (1989). PO_2 chemoreception in arterial chemoreceptors. *Annu. Rev. Physiol., 51,* 835–844.

Adachi, A., Niijima, A., & Jacobs, H. L. (1976). An hepatic osmoreceptor mechanism in the rat: Electrophysiological and behavioral studies. *Am. J. Physiol., 231,* 1043–1049.

Ádám, G. (1967). *Interoception and behaviour. An experimental study*. Budapest: Akadémiai Kiadó.

Ádám, G. (1974). Interoceptive stimuli and learning (Toward a "psychophysics" of visceroception). *Proc. International Union of Physiological Sciences* (Vol. 10). New Delhi: Core Book Programme of the Government of India.

Ádám, G. (1978). Visceroception, awareness and behavior. In G. E. Schwartz & D. Shapiro (Eds.), *Consciousness and self-regulation* (Vol. 2, pp. 199–213). New York: Plenum Press.

Ádám, G. (1980). *Perception, consciousness, memory. Reflections of a biologist*. Budapest/New York: Akadémiai Kiadó/Plenum Press.

Ádám, G. (1983). Intestinal afferent influence on behavior. In R. Hölzl & W. E. Whitehead (Eds.), *Psychophysiology of the gastrointestinal tract* (pp. 351–360). New York: Plenum Press.

Ádám, G. (1993). Viscerosensory functions. In B. Smith & G. Adelman (Eds.), *Neuroscience Year Supplement 3 to the Encyclopedia of neuroscience*. Boston, Basel, Berlin: Birkhäuser.

215

Ádám, G., Balázs, L., Vidos, T., & Keszler, P. (1990). Detection of colon distension in colonostomy patients. *Psychophysiology, 27,* 451–456.

Ádám, G., Bárdos, G., Hoffmann, I., & Nagy, K. (1977). Hemispheric lateralization of visceroceptive influence on operant behavior. In *Proc. IUPS. (Vol. XI).* Paris: Comité Natl. Franc. Sci. Physiol.

Ádám, G., & Mészáros, I. (1957). Contributions to the higher nervous connections of the renal pelvis and the ureter. *Acta Physiol. Hung., 12,* 327.

Ádám, G., Mészáros, I., Lehotzky, K., & Kelemen, V. (1960). On the differentiation of an interoceptive conditioned arousal reaction. *Electroencephalogr. Clin. Neurophysiol., 12,* 935.

Ádám, G., Mészáros, I., & Zubor, L. (1957). On the joint function of the cerebral hemispheres in connection with renal pelvic and ureteral symmetric afferent impulses. *Acta Physiol. Hung., 12,* 335.

Ádám, G., Preisich, P., Kukorelli, T., & Kelemen, V. (1965). Changes in human cerebral electrical activity in response to mechanical stimulation of the duodenum. *Electroencephalogr. Clin. Neurophysiol., 18,* 409.

Adrian, E. D. (1933). Afferent impulses in the vagus and their effect on respiration. *J. Physiol. (London), 79,* 332.

Agostoni, E., Chinnock, J. E., Daly De Burgh, M., & Murray, J. G. (1957). Functional and histological studies on the vagus nerve and its branches to heart, lunes and abdominal viscera in the cat. *J. Physiol. (London), 135,* 182–205.

Airapetyants, E. S. (1952). *Higher nervous activity and the receptors of the internal organs* [in Russian]. Moscow: Publishing House of the Academy of Science of the USSR.

Andrews, P. L.R. (1986). Vagal afferent innervation of the gastrointestinal tract. In F. Cervero & J. F. B. Morrison (Eds.), *Visceral sensation* (pp. 65–86). Amsterdam: Elsevier.

Anokhin, P. K. (1968). *The biology and the neurophysiology of the conditioned reflex* [in Russian]. Moscow: Publishing House of the Academy of Sciences of the USSR.

Aristotle. (1982). *Rétorika* [Hungarian translation from the Greek original by Tamás Adamik]. Budapest: Gondolat.

Aviado, D. M., & Schmidt, C. F. (1955). Reflexes from stretch receptors in blood vessels, heart and lungs. *Physiol. Rev., 35,* 247.

Bainbridge, F. A. (1914). On some cardiac reflexes. *J. Physiol. (London), 48,* 332.

Bárdos, G. (1989). Behavioral consequences of intestinal distension: Aversivity and discomfort. *Physiol. Behav., 45,* 79–85.

Bárdos, G., & Ádám, G. (1978). Visceroceptive control of operant behavior in rats. *Physiol. Behav., 20,* 369–375.

Bárdos, G., & Ádám, G. (1980). Complex studies of the effects of visceroceptive stimulation on the behavior of the rat. In R. Sinz & M. R. Rosenzweig (Eds.), *Psychophysiology 1980* (pp. 219–223). Jena: Amsterdam. Gustav Fischer-Verlag/Elsevier.

Bárdos, G., Nagy, J., & Ádám, G. (1980). Thresholds of behavioral reactions evoked by intestinal and skin stimuli in rats. *Physiol. Behav., 24*, 661–665.

Barlett, F. C. (1932). *Remembering*. London: Cambridge University Press.

Barnard, J. W. (1936). A phylogenetic study of the visceral afferent areas associated with the facial, glossopharyngeal, and vagus nerves, and their fiber connections, the efferent facial nucleus. *J. Comp. Neurol., 65*, 503.

Békésy, G. von. (1947). A new audiometer. *Acta Oto-Laryngol., 35*, 411–422.

Beller, N. N. (1954). The influence of gravidity on the chemoreceptors of the ovaries [in Russian]. *Bull. Exp. Biol. Med., 37*, 8.

Benussi, V. (1914). Gesetze der inadäquaten Gestaltauffassung. *Arch. gesamte Psychol., 32*, 417.

Bergson, H. (1914). *Le Rire*. Paris: Félix Alcan.

Bessou, P., & Perl, E. R. (1966). A movement receptor in the small intestine. *J. Physiol. (London), 182*, 404–426.

Blough, D. S. (1961). Experiments in animal psychophysics. *Sci. Am., 205*, 113–122.

Boenko, I. D. (1950). *Materials on the physiology of thermoreceptors* [in Russian]. Dissertation, Sverdlovsk.

Bradley, L. A., & Richter, J. E. (1996). Esophageal disorders and their relationship to psychiatric disease. In K. W. Olden (Ed.), *Handbook of functional gastrointestinal disorders* (pp. 145–171). New York: Dekker.

Brener, J., & Jones, J. M. (1974). Interoceptive discrimination in intact humans: Detection of cardiac activity. *Physiol. Behav., 13*, 763–767.

Broadbent, D. E. (1958). *Perception and communication*. New York: Pergamon.

Bykov, K. M. (1947). *The cerebral cortex and the internal organs* (2nd ed.) [in Russian]. Moscow: Medgiz.

Cabanac, M. (1971). Physiological role of pleasure. *Science, 173*, 1103–1107.

Cannon, W. B. (1929). *Bodily changes in pain, hunger, fear and rage*. New York: Appleton.

Cannon, W. B., and Washburn, A. L. (1912). An exploration of hunger. *Am. J. Physiol., 29*, 441–454.

Cervero, F., & Foreman, R. D. (1990). Sensory innervation of the viscera. In A. D. Loewy & K. M. Spyer (Eds.), *Central regulation of autonomic functions* (pp. 104–125). London: Oxford University Press.

Cervero, F., & Morrison, J. F. B. (Eds.). (1986). *Visceral sensation. Progress in Brain Research* (Vol. 67). Amsterdam: Elsevier.

Cervero, F., & Sharkey, K. A. (1988). An electrophysiological and anatomical study of intestinal afferent fibers in the rat. *J. Physiol. (London), 401*, 361–380.

Charcot, J.-M. (1888–1894). *Oevres complètes* (Vols. 1–9). Paris: Delahaye et Lecrosnier.

Chernigovski, V. N. (1960). *The interoceptors* [in Russian]. Moscow: Medgiz.

Clarke, G. D., & Davison, J. S. (1978). Mucosal receptors in the gastric antrum and small intestine of the rat with afferent fibers in the cervical vagus. *J. Physiol. (London), 284*, 55–67.

Cook, I. J., Van Eeden, A., & Collins, S. M. (1987). Patients with irritable bowel syndrome have greater pain tolerance than normal subjects. *Gastroenterology, 93,* 727–733.

Cyon, E. D., & Ludwig, C. (1866). Die Reflexe eines der sensibilen Nerven des Herzens auf der Motorischen der Blutgefässe. *Berichte Sächs. Ges. Wiss., 18,* 307.

Danilewsky, V. (1875). Experimentelle beiträge zur Physiologie des Gehirns. *Pflügers Arch. Gesamte Physiol., 11,* 128.

Darwin, C. R. (1872). *The expression of emotions in man and animals.* London: John Murray.

Davison, J. S., & Clarke, G. D. (1988). Mechanical properties and sensitivity to CCK of vagal gastric slowly adapting mechanoreceptors. *Am. J. Physiol., 255,* G55–G61.

De Castro, F. (1928). Sur la structure et l'innervation du sinus carotidien de l'homme et des mammifères. *Trav. Lab. Invest. Biol. Univ. Madrid, 25,* 331.

De Groat, W. C. (1986). Spinal cord projections and neuropeptides in visceral afferent neurons. In F. Cervero & J. F. B. Morrison (Eds.), *Visceral sensation* (pp. 165–187). Amsterdam: Elsevier.

Dell, P. (1952). Corrélations entre le système nerveux végétatif et le système de la vie de relation. *J. Physiol. (Paris), 44,* 471.

Delov, V. E. (1949). Materials on the electrophysiological characteristics of cortico-visceral interrelations [in Russian]. *Tr. Voenno-Med. Acad., 17,* 117.

Dixon, N. (1981). *Preconscious processing.* New York: Wiley.

Dogiel, A. (1878). Zur Kenntnis der Nerven der Ureteren. *Arch. Mikrosk. Anat., 15,* 64.

Drossman, D. A., Grant Thompson, W., Talley, N. J., Funch-Jensen, P., Janssens, J., & Whitehead, W. E. (1990). Identification of sub-groups of functional gastrointestinal disorders. *Gastroenterol. Int., 3,* 159–172.

Duval, S., & Wicklund, R. A. (1972). *A theory of objective self-awareness.* New York: Academic Press.

Dworkin, B. R. (1993). *Learning and physiological regulation.* Chicago: University of Chicago Press.

Dworkin, B. R., Filewich, R. J., Miller, N. E., Craigmyle, N., & Pickering, T. G. (1979). Baroreceptor activation reduces reactivity to noxious stimulation: Implications for hypertension. *Science, 205,* 1299–1301.

Ehrenfels, C. von. (1890). Über Gestaltqualitäten. *Vierteljahresrschr. Wiss. Philos., 14,* 249–263, 285–292.

El Ouzzani, T., & Mei, N. (1981). Acido- et glucorécepteurs vagaux de la région gastro-duodénale. *Exp. Brain Res., 42,* 442–452.

El Ouzzani, T., & Mei, N. (1982). Electrophysiological properties and role of the vagal thermoreceptors of lower esophagus and stomach of cat. *Gastroenterology, 83,* 995–1002.

Evans, D. H.L., & Murray, J. G. (1954). Histological and functional studies on the fibre composition of the vagus nerve of the rabbit. *J. Anat., 88,* 320–337.

Fechner, G. T. (1966). *Elements of psychophysics*. New York: Holt, Rinehart & Winston. (Original work published 1860).

Fent, J., Balázs, L., Buzás, G., Erasmus, P. L., Hölzl, R., Kovács, Á., Weisz, J., & Ádám, G. (1998). Colonic sensitivity in irritable bowel syndrome and normal subjects according to their hemispheric preference and cognitive style. *Int. Physiol. Behav. Sci.* (submitted).

Fillenz, M., & Widdicombe, J. G. (1972). Receptors of the lungs and airways. In E. Neil (Ed.), *Enteroceptors* (pp. 81–112). Berlin: Springer.

Firth, R. (1974). Sense experience. In E. C. Carterre & M. P. Friedman (Eds.), *Handbook of perception* (Vol. 1, pp. 3–18). New York: Academic Press.

Floyd, K., Hick, V. E., Koley, J., & Morrison, J. F. B. (1977). The effect of bradykinin on afferent unit in intraabdominal symphathetic nerve trunks. *Q. J. Exp. Physiol., 62,* 19–36.

Freeman, W. J. (1981). A physiological hypothesis on perception. *Perspect. Biol. Med., 24,* 561–592.

Freeman, W. J. (1983). The physiology of mental images. Academic address. *Biol. Psychiatry, 18,* 1107–1125.

Freud, S. (1964). *New introductory lectures on psychoanalysis*. New York: Norton. (Original work published 1933).

Gambashidze, S. K. (1951). *Materials on the physiology of interoceptors of the sexual sphere* [in Russian]. Tbilisi: Gruzmedgiz.

Garcia, J., Hankins, W. G., & Rusiniak, K. W. (1974). Behavioral regulation of the milieu interne in man and rat. *Science, 185,* 824–831.

Ghiselin, M. T. (1969). *The triumph of Darwinian method*. Berkeley: University of California Press.

Gibson, J. J. (1979). *The ecological approach to visual perception*. Boston: Houghton Mifflin.

Granit, R. (1955). *Receptors and sensory perception*. New Haven, CT: Yale University Press.

Gray, J. A. B. (1959). Initiation of impulses at receptors. In *Handbook of physiology* (Vol. 1, p. 123). Washington, DC: American Physiological Society.

Green, D. M., & Swets, J. (1966). *Signal detection theory and psychophysics*. New York: Wiley.

Gregory, R. L. (1974). Choosing a paradigm for perception. In E. C. Carterre & M. P. Friedman (Eds.), *Handbook of perception* (Vol. 2, pp. 255–284). New York: Academic Press.

Hajduczok, G., Chapleau, M. W., & Abboud, F. M. (1988). Rheoreceptors in the carotid sinus of dog. *Proc. Natl. Acad. Sci. USA, 85,* 7399–7403.

Haller, A. (1764). *Elementa physiologica*. Lausanne.

Hantas, M. N., Katkin, E. S., & Reed, S. D. (1984). Cerebral lateralization and heartbeat discrimination. *Psychophysiology, 21,* 274–278.

Hardcastle, J., Hardcastle, P. T., & Sanford, P. A. (1978). Effect of actively transported hexoses on afferent nerve discharge from rat small intestine. *J. Physiol. (London), 285,* 71–84.

Harding, R., & Leek, B. F. (1972). Gastro-duodenal receptor responses to chemical and mechanical stimuli, investigated by a single fiber technique. *J. Physiol. (London)*, *222*, 139–140.

Hartmann, E. von. (1884). *Philosophy of the unconscious.* Strasbourg: Trübner.

Head, H. (1920). *Studies in neurology* (2 vols.). London: Oxford Medical Publishers.

Hebb, D. O. (1949). *The organization of behavior.* New York: Wiley.

Heger, P. (1887). Einige Versuche über die Empfindlichkeit der Gefässe. *Ludwig Beitr. Physiol.*, *193*, 61–66.

Hering, H. E. (1923). Die Karotisdruckversuche. *Münch. Med. Wochenschr.*, *70*, 1287.

Hering, E., & Breuer, I. (1868). Die Sebsteuerung der Atmung durch den Nervus Vagus. *B. Akad. Wiss. Wien*, *57–58*, 672, 909.

Heymans, C. (1950). Chemoreceptors and regulation of respiration. *Acta Physiol. Scand.*, *22*, 1.

Heymans, C., & Neil, E. (1958). *Reflexogenic areas of the cardiovascular system.* London: Churchill.

Hilgard, E. (1965). *Hypnotic susceptibility.* New York: Harcourt, Brace & World.

Hölzl, R., Erasmus, L. P., & Möltner, A. (1996). Detection, discrimination and sensation of visceral stimuli. *Biol. Psychol.*, *42*, 199–214.

Hölzl, R., Möltner, A., Erasmus, L. P., Samaj, S., Waldmann, H. C., & Neidig, C. W. (1994). *Detection, discrimination and sensation of visceral stimuli.* Forschungsberichte aus dem Otto-Selz-Institut. No. 30. University of Mannheim.

Hubel, D. H., & Wiesel, T. N. (1963). Receptive fields of cells in striate cortex of very young visually inexperienced kittens. *J. Neurophysiol.*, *26*, 994–1002.

Iggo, A. (1955). Tension receptors in the stomach and the urinary bladder. *J. Physiol. (London)*, *128*, 593–607.

Iggo, A. (1957a). Gastro-intestinal tension receptors with unmyelinated afferent fibers in the vagus of the cat. *Q. J. Exp. Physiol.*, *42*, 130–141.

Iggo, A. (1957b). Gastric mucosal chemoreceptors with vagal afferent fibers in the cat. *Q. J. Exp. Physiol.*, *42*, 398–409.

Iggo, A. (1986). Afferent C-fibres and visceral sensation. In F. Cervero & J. F. B. Morrison (Eds.), *Visceral sensation* (pp. 29–48). Amsterdam: Elsevier.

James, W. (1907). *Psychology.* New York: Henry Holt.

Janet, P. (1914–1915). Psychoanalysis. *J. Abnorm. Psychol.*, *9*, 1–35, 153–187.

Jänig, W. (1996). Neurobiology of visceral afferent neurons: Neuroanatomy, functions, organ regulations and sensations. *Biol. Psychol.*, *42*, 29–51.

Jänig, W., & Morrison, J. F. B. (1986). Functional properties of visceral afferent neurons supplying abdominal and pelvic organs with special emphasis on visceral nociception. In F. Cervero & J. F. B. Morrison (Eds.), *Visceral sensation* (pp. 87–114). Amsterdam: Elsevier.

Jeannigros, R., & Mei, N. (1980). Données préliminaires sur la réponse des chémorécepteurs intestinaux aux acides aminés. *Reprod. Nutr. Dev.*, *20*, 1615–1619.

Jones, G. E. (1994). Perception of visceral sensations. In P. K. Ackles, J. R. Jennings, & M. G. H. Coles (Eds.), *Advances in psychophysiology* (Vol. 5, pp. 55–192). Greenwich, CT: JAI Press.

Julesz, B. (1987). Texture perception. In G. Adelman (Ed.), *Encyclopedia of neuroscience* (Vol. 2, pp. 1200–1202). Boston Basel: Birkhäuser.

Katkin, E. S. (1985). Blood, sweat and tears: Individual differences in autonomic self-perception. *Psychophysiology, 22,* 125–137.

Kimura, D. (1961). Cerebral dominance and perception of verbal stimuli. *Can. J. Psychol., 15,* 166–171.

Kline, E. M., & Bidder, T. G. (1946). A study of the subjective sensations associated with extrasystoles. *Am. Heart J., 31,* 254–259.

Koch, E. (1932). Die Irradiation der Pressorezeptorischen Kreislaufreflexe. *Klin. Wochenschr., 11,* 225.

Köhler, W. (1925). *The mentality of apes.* New York: Harcourt, Brace.

Kolosov, N. G. (1954). *The innervation of the internal organs and of the cardiovascular system.* Moscow: Publishing House of the Academy of Sciences of the USSR.

Koshtoyants, H. S. (1950–1957). *Foundations of comparative physiology* (in Russian) (Vols. 1 and 2). Moscow: Publishing House of the Academy of Sciences of the USSR.

Kravchinski, B. D. (1945). The evolution of the reflex connections of the respiratory centers of vertebrates [in Russian]. *Fiziol. Zh. Sechenova, 31,* 11.

Kuhn, T. S. (1970). *The structure of scientific revolution* (2nd ed.). Chicago: University of Chicago Press.

Kukorelli, T., Ádám, G., Gimes, R., & Tóth, F. (1972). Uteral stimulation and vigilance level in humans. *Acta Physiol. Hung., 42,* 403–410.

Kukorelli, T., & Détári, L. (1994). Effects of viscerosensory stimulation on hypothalamically elicited predatory behavior in cats. *Physiol. Behav., 55,* 705–710.

Kukorelli, T., & Juhász, G. (1976). Electroencephalographic synchronization induced by stimulation of small intestine and splanchnic nerve in cats. *Electroencephalogr. Clin. Neurophysiol., 41,* 491–500.

Kukorelli, T., & Juhász, G. (1983). Tonic and phasic modifications of viscerosensory evoked potentials during sleep in cats. *Acta Physiol. Hung., 61,* 237–246.

Kumazava, T. (1986). Sensory innervation of reproductive organs. In F. Cervero & J. F. B. Morrison (Eds.), *Visceral sensation* (pp. 115–131). Amsterdam: Elsevier.

Lacey, B. C., & Lacey, J. I. (1978). Two-way communication between the heart and the brain: Significance of time within the cardiac cycle. *Am. Psychol., 33,* 99–113.

Lange, C. G. (1905). *Les émotions. Étude psycho-physiologique.* Paris: Félix Alcan.

Langley, J. N. (1903). The autonomic nervous system. *Brain, 26,* 1–26.

Langley, J. N. (1922). *Das Autonome Nervensystem.* Berlin: Springer-Verlag.

Langley, J. N., & Dickinson, W. L. (1889). On the local paralysis of peripheral ganglia, and on the connexion of different classes of nerve fibers with them. *Proc. R. Soc. London, 46,* 423–431.

Lavrentiev, V. I. (1948). Sensory innervation of internal organs. In *Morphology of sensory innervation of internal organs* [in Russian]. Moscow: Publishing House of the Academy of Sciences of the USSR.

Lebedeva, V. A., & Khayutin, V. M. (1952). The reflexes from the chemoreceptors of the urinary bladder. In *Problems of physiology of interoception* [in Russian]. Moscow: Publishing House of the Academy of Sciences of the USSR.

Leek, B. F. (1972). Abdominal visceral receptors. In E. Neile (Ed.), *Enteroceptors* (pp. 113–160) . Berlin: Springer.

Leek, B. F. (1977). Abdominal and pelvic visceral receptors. *Br. Med. Bull., 33,* 163–168.

Leibniz, G. W. (1765). Nouveaux essais sur l'entendement humaine. In R. E. Raspe (Ed.), *Oevres Philosophiques de feu M Leibnitz.* Leipzig: Schreuder.

Leventhal, H., Meyer, D., & Nerenz, D. (1980). The common sense representation of illness danger. In S. Rachman (Ed.), *Medical psychology* (Vol. 2, pp. 116–153). New York: Pergamon.

Lintvarev, S. I. (1901). *The role of fats in the transit of food from the stomach in the gut* [in Russian]. Dissertation, Saint Petersburg.

Lipps, T. (1897). Raumaesthetik und geometrischoptische Täuschungen. *Schriftenr. Ges. Psychol. Forsch. 2.*

Lovatt Evans, C. (1949). *Principles of human physiology* [Originally written by E. H. Starling] (10th ed.). London: Churchill.

Mandler, G., Mandler, J. M., and Noiller, E. T. (1958). Autonomic feedback: The perception of autonomic activity. *J. Abnormal Soc. Psychol., 56,* 367–373.

Manning, A. P., Thompson, W. G., Heaton, K. W., & Morris, A. F. (1978). Toward positive diagnosis of the irritable bowel. *Br. Med. J., II,* 653–654.

Mason, R. E. (1961). *Internal perception and bodily functioning.* New York: International Universities Press.

Mayer, E. A., & Gebhart, G. F. (1994). Basic and clinical aspects of visceral hyperalgesia. *Gastroenterology, 107,* 271–293.

McFarland, R. A. (1975). Heart rate perception and heart rate control. *Psychophysiology, 12,* 402–405.

Mechanic, D. (1972). Social psychological factors affecting the presentation of bodily complaints. *New Engl. J. Med., 286,* 1132–1139.

Mei, N. (1978). Vagal glucoreceptors in the small intestine of the cat. *J. Physiol. (London), 282,* 485–506.

Mei, N. (1983). Sensory structures in the viscera. In D. Ottoson (Ed.), *Progress in sensory physiology* (Vol. 4, pp. 1–42). Berlin: Springer-Verlag.

Mei, N. (1990). Les troubles de la sensibilité intestinale et le syndrome de l'intestin irritable. *Gastroenterol. Clin. Biol., 14,* 29C–32C.

Meunier, P. (1990). L'intestin hypersensible. *Gastroenterol. Clin. Biol., 14,* 33C–36C.

Miller, N. E. (1971). *Selected papers.* New York: Aldine–Atherton.

Milner, B., Taylor, L., & Sperry, W. R. (1968). Lateralized suppression of dichotically presented digits after commissural section in man. *Science, 161,* 184–186.

Milohin, A. A. (1963). *The interoceptors of the alimentary tract of some higher vertebrates* [in Russian]. Moscow: Publishing House of the Academy of Sciences of the USSR.

Minut-Sorokhtina, O. P., & Sirotin, B. V. (1957). *The physiological importance of the venous receptors* [in Russian]. Moscow: Medgiz.

Mishkin, M., & Appenzeller, T. (1987). The anatomy of memory. *Sci. Am., 256,* 80–89.

Moiseeva, N. A. (1952). On interoceptive reflexes in the embryogenesis [in Russian]. *Dokl. Akad. Nauk SSSR, 37,* 321.

Montgomery, W. A., & Jones, G. E. (1984). Laterality, emotionality and heartbeat perception. *Psychophysiology, 21,* 459–465.

Mountcastle, V. B. (1975). The view from within: Pathways to the study of perception. *Johns Hopkins Med. J., 136,* 109–131.

Mountcastle, V. B. (1980). Sensory receptors and neural encoding: Introduction to sensory processes. In *Medical physiology* (14th ed., chapter 11). St. Louis: Mosby.

Mountcastle, V. (1987). Representations and the construction of reality. The Gordon Wilson lecture. In *Transactions of the American Clinical and Climatological Association* (Vol. 99, pp. 70–90). Baltimore: Johns Hopkins University Press.

Müller, J. (1840). *Handbuch der Physiologie der Menschen für Vorlesungen.* Koblenz: J. Holscher.

Neafsey, E. J. (1990). Prefrontal cortical control of the autonomic nervous system: Anatomical and physiological observations. *Prog. Brain Res., 85,* 147–166.

Neil, E., Ström, L., & Zotterman, Y. (1950). Action potential studies of afferent fibers in the IXth and Xth cranial nerves of the frog. *Acta Physiol. Scand., 20,* 338.

Neumann, A. (1906). Über die Temperatur Empfindlichkeit des Magens. *Wien. Klin. Wocehnschr., 30,* 923.

Newman, P. P. (1974). *Visceral afferent functions of the nervous system.* London: Edward Arnold.

Niculescu, I. (1958). *Morphological aspects of visceral nerve endings* [in Romanian]. Bucharest: Editura Medicala.

Niijima, A. (1969). Afferent impulse discharges from glucoreceptors in the liver of the guinea pig. *Ann. N.Y. Acad. Sci., 157,* 690–700.

Niijima, A. (1971). Afferent discharges from arterial mechanoreceptors in the kidney of the rabbit. *J. Physiol. (London), 219,* 477–485.

Nikiforovsky, P. (1913). On depressor nerve fibers in the vagus of the frog. *J. Physiol. (London), 45,* 459.

Nisbett, R. E., & Wilson, T. D. (1977). Telling more than we can know: Verbal reports on mental processes. *Psychol. Rev., 84,* 231–259.

Pagano, G. (1900). Sur la sensibilité du coeur et des vaisseaux sanguins. *Arch. Ital. Biol., 33,* 1.

Paintal, A. S. (1953). A study of right and left atrial receptors. *J. Physiol. (London), 120,* 596.

Paintal, A. S. (1954). A study of gastric stretch receptors, their role in the peripheral mechanism of satiation of hunger and thirst. *J. Physiol. (London), 126*, 255.

Paintal, A. S. (1969). Mechanism of stimulation of type-J pulmonary receptors. *J. Physiol. (London), 203*, 511–532.

Paintal, A. S. (1973). Vagal sensory receptors and their reflex effects. *Physiol. Rev., 53*, 159–227.

Paintal, A. S. (1986). The visceral sensations: Some basic mechanisms. In F. Cervero & J. F. B. Morrison (Eds.), *Visceral sensation*. Amsterdam: Elsevier.

Pavlov, I. P. (1951–1954). *Complete works in 6 volumes* [in Russian]. Moscow: Publishing House of the Academy of Sciences of the USSR.

Pennebaker, J. W. (1982). *The psychology of physical symptoms*. Berlin: Springer.

Pennebaker, J. W. (1995). Beyond laboratory-based cardiac perception: Ecological interoception. In D. Vaitl & R. Schandry (Eds.), *From the heart to the brain* (pp. 389–406). Frankfurt am Main: Peter Lang Verlag.

Piaget, J. (1937–1954). *The construction of reality in the child*. New York: Basic Books.

Pischinger, A. (1934). Über die Entwicklung und das Wesen des Carotislabyrinths bei Anuren. *Z. Anat. Entwicklungsgesch., 103*, 547.

Plato. (1899–1907). Charmides. In J. Burnet (Ed.), *Platonis opera* (Vol. 5, 1st ed.). London: Oxford University Press.

Polányi, M. (1964). *Personal knowledge: Toward a post-critical philosophy*. New York: Harper.

Pribram, K. (1971). *Languages of the brain*. Englewood Cliffs, NJ: Prentice–Hall.

Ramón y Cajal, S. (1909). *Histologie du système nerveux de l'homme et des vertébrés*. Paris: Maloine.

Rawson, S. W., & Quick, K. P. (1972). Localisation of intra-abdominal thermoreceptors in the ewe. *J. Physiol. (London), 222*, 665–677.

Recordati, G. M., Moss, N. G., Genovesi, S., & Rogenes, P. T. (1980). Renal receptors in the rat sensitive to chemical alterations of their environment. *Circ. Res., 46*, 395–405.

Reinhold, K. L. (1789). *Attempt at a new theory of human ideation*. Jena: Fischer.

Révész, G. (1928). *Über taktile Agnosie*. Haarlem: De Erven F. Boon.

Révész, G. (1934). System der optischen und haptischen Raumtäuschungen. *Z. Psychol., 131*, 7.

Révész, G. (1956). *Optik und Haptik* (Posthumous ed.). Berlin: Springer-Verlag.

Schachter, S., and Singer, J. (1962). Cognitive, social, and psychological determinants of emotional state. *Psychol. Rev., 69*, 379–399.

Schandry, R., & Montoya, P. (1996). Event-related brain potentials and the processing of cardiac activity. *Biol. Psychol., 42*, 75–85.

Schandry, R., & Specht, G. (1981). The influence of psychological and physical stress on the perception of heartbeats. *Psychophysiology, 18*, 154.

Schofield, G. C. (1960). Experimental studies on the innervation of the mucous membrane of the gut. *Brain, 83*, 490–514.

Schopenhauer, A. (1844). *Die Welt als Wille und Vorstellung*. Leipzig: Brockhaus.

Schumann, F. (1900). Beiträge zur Analyse der Gesichtswahrnemungen. *Z. Psychol.*, *23*, 1–32; 24, 1–33.

Schwiegk, H. (1935). Der Lungenentastungreflex. *Pflügers Arch. Gesamte. Physiol.*, *326*, 206.

Sechenov, I. M. (1935). *The reflexes of the brain* [in Russian]. Leningrad: Publisher of the Institute of Experimental Medicine.

Senden, M. Von. (1960). *Space and sight* (P. Heath, Trans.). London: Methuen. (Original work published 1932)

Serdyukov, A. S. (1899). *One of the main conditions of the transit of food from the stomach into the gut* [in Russian]. Dissertation, Saint Petersburg.

Sharma, K. N., & Nasset, E. S. (1962). Electrical activity in mesenteric nerves after perfusion of gut lumen. *Am. J. Physiol.*, *202*, 725–730.

Sherrington, C. S. (1899). Marshall Hall Address. *Med. Chir. Trans.*, *82*.

Sherrington, C. S. (1911). *The integrative action of the nervous system.* London: Constable.

Simanovski, N. P. (1881). *On the problem of the stimulation of sensory nerves on the regulation and nutrition of the heart* [in Russian] Dissertation, Saint Petersburg.

Skinner, B. F. (1938). *The behavior of organisms.* New York: Appleton–Century–Crofts.

Slucki, H., Ádám, G., & Porter, R. W. (1965). Operant discrimination of an interoceptive stimulus in rhesus monkeys. *J. Exp. Anal. Behav.*, *8*, 405.

Snowdon, C. T. (1970). Gastrointestinal sensory and motor control of food intake. *J. Comp. Physiol. Psychol.*, *71*, 68–76.

Sokolov, E. N. (1963). Higher nervous functions: The orienting reflex. *Annu. Rev. Physiol.*, *25*, 545–580.

Sokolov, V. A. (1955). *On the characteristics of internal analyzers of the fish* [in Russian]. Dissertation, Leningrad.

Spencer, H. (1897). *Principles of psychology.* New York: Appleton.

Sperry, R. W. (1977). Forebrain commissurotomy and conscious awareness. *J. Med. Philos.*, *2*, 101–126.

Spinoza, B. (1677). *How to improve your mind* (R. H. M. Elwes, Trans.). New York: Wisdom Library (1956).

Stern, R. M., Ray, W. J., & Davis, C. M. (1980). *Psycho-physiological recording.* London: Oxford University Press.

Stevens, S. S. (1975). *Psychophysics: Introduction to its perceptual, neural and social prospects.* New York: Wiley.

Stevens, S. S. (1979). Psychophysics. In H. J. Eysensk, W. Arnold, & R. Meili (Eds.), *Encyclopedia of psychology* (pp. 867–871). New York: Seabury Press.

Strazhenko, N. D. (1904). *On the physiology of the gut* [in Russian].Dissertation, Saint Petersburg.

Stunkard, A., and Koch, C. (1964). The interpretation of gastric motility. *Arch. Gen. Psychiatry, 11*, 74–82.

Swets, J. A. (Ed.). (1964). *Signal detection and recognition by human observers*. New York: Wiley.

Thorndike, E. L. (1898). Animal intelligence. *Psychol. Monogr., 2*(8).

Trabant, J. (Ed.) (1996). *Origins of language*. Budapest: Collegium Budapest, Institute for Advanced Study.

Vaitl, D. (1996). Interoception. *Biol. Psychol., 42*, 1–27.

Vaitl, D., & Schandry, R. (Eds.) (1995). *From the heart to the brain. The psychophysiology of circulation–brain interaction*. Frankfurt am Main: Peter Lang Verlag.

Valbo, A. B., & Johanson, R. S. (1984). Properties of cutaneous mechanoreceptors in the human hand related to touch sensation. *Hum. Neurobiol., 3*, 3.

Verney, E. B. (1946). Absorption and excretion of water: Antidiuretic hormone. *Lancet, 251*, 739.

Vygotsky, L. S. (1960). *The development of higher mental functions* [in Russian]. Moscow: Medgiz.

Weddell, G. (1941). The multiple innervation of sensory spots in the skin. *J. Anat., 75*, 441.

Weiskrantz, L. (1986). *Blindsight. A case study and implications*. London: Oxford University Press.

Weisz, J., & Ádám, G. (1993). Hemispheric preference and lateral eye movements evoked by bilateral visual stimuli. *Neuropsychologia, 31*, 1299–1306.

Weisz, J., & Ádám, G. (1996). The influence of cardiac phase on reaction time depending on heart period length and on stimulus and response laterality. *Psychobiology, 24*, 169–175.

Weisz, J., Balázs, L., & Ádám, G. (1988). The influence of self-focused attention on heartbeat perception. *Psychophysiology, 25*, 193–199.

Weisz, J., Balázs, L., & Ádám, G. (1994). The effect of monocular viewing on heartbeat discrimination. *Psychophysiology, 31*, 370–374.

Weisz, J., Balázs, L., Láng, E., & Ádám, G. (1990). The effect of lateral visual fixation and the direction of eye movements on heartbeat discrimination. *Psychophysiology, 27*, 523–527.

Weisz, J., Soroker, N., Oksenberg, A., & Myslobodsky, M. S. (1995). Effect of hemi-thalamic damage on K-complexes evoked by monaural stimuli during midafternoon sleep. *Electroencephalogr. Clin. Neurophysiol., 94*, 148–150.

Weisz, J., Szilágyi, N., Láng, E., & Ádám, G. (1992). The influence of monocular viewing on heart period variability. *Int. J. Psychophysiol., 12*, 11–18.

Whitehead, W. E. (1983). Interoception. In R. Hölzl & W. E. Whitehead (Eds.), *Psychophysiology of the gastrointestinal tract* (pp. 333–350). New York: Plenum Press.

Whitehead, W. E., Drescher, V. M., Heiman, P., & Blackwell, B. (1977). Relation of heart rate control to heartbeat perception. *Biofeedback Self-regul., 2*, 371–392.

Whitteridge, D. (1948). Afferent nerve fibers from the heart and lungs in the cervical vagus. *J. Physiol. (London), 107*, 496.

Whyte, L. L. (1960). *The unconscious before Freud*. New York: Basic Books.

Wicklund, R. A. (1978). Objective self-awareness. In L. Berkowitz (Ed.), *Cognitive theories in social psychology.* New York: Academic Press.

Widdicombe, J. G. (1954). Receptors in the trachea and bronchi of the cat. *J. Physiol. (London),* 123, 7.

Yost, R. M. (1974). Some philosophical problems of perception. In E. C. Carterre & M. P. Friedman (Eds.), *Handbook of perception* (Vol. 1, pp. 19–39). New York: Academic Press.

Zamyatina, O. N. (1954). Electrophysiological characteristics and functional importance of the afferent impulses from the receptors of the intestinal wall [in Russian]. *Tr. Inst. Fiziol., 111,* 193.

Zotterman, Y. (1953). Special senses: Thermal receptors. *Annu. Rev. Physiol., 15,* 357.

Index

Note to the reader: Appendixes I–III are not included in this Index.

229